Doctor, Why Do I Hurt So Much?

How to Combat Your Arthritis or Arthritis-Like Condition and Start Enjoying an Active Life

Second Edition

Mark H. Greenberg, MD, FACR, RMSK, RhMSUS
Nathan Wei, MD, FACP, FACR

This book is not meant to replace your doctor. It is an aid to help you and your doctor reach an accurate diagnosis. It should not be used to provide or encourage self-diagnosis. Treatment recommendations in the book should serve as only a guide. All medical diagnosis and subsequent treatments are to be undertaken only by a qualified physician.

Doctor, Why Do I Hurt So Much? How to Combat Your Arthritis or Arthritis-Like Condition and Start Enjoying an Active Life.

Library of Congress Cataloging-in-Publication Data
Greenberg, Mark H.

Doctor, why do I hurt so much? How to combat your arthritis or arthritis-like-condition and start enjoying an active life / Mark H. Greenberg. cm. Includes index. ISBN 13: 978-1543185225, ISBN 10: 1543185223 $11.95 1. Arthritis—Popular works, 2. Rheumatism—Popular works.
II. Title.

RC933.G64 1992
616.772—dc20

92-3352
CIP

Printed in the United States of America
10 9 8 7 6 5 4 3 2 1

Dedication

To my wife, Brenda. The woman that I have
been waiting for.

Mark Greenberg

To my wife, Judy. My Best Friend.

Nathan Wei

Table of Contents

About the Authors

Mark H. Greenberg, MD, FACR, RMSK, RhMSUS earned his M.D. degree from Northwestern University Medical School, Chicago, Illinois. After completing his fellowship in rheumatology in 1984 at Albert Einstein-Montefiore Medical Center, New York City, Dr. Greenberg began practice in Port St. Lucie, Florida. His articles have appeared in the *Journal of the American Academy of Dermatology,* the *Journal of Rheumatology,* the *Journal of Clinical Investigation,* and the *Journal of the American Academy of Disability Evaluating Physicians.* He practices rheumatology, internal medicine, and musculoskeletal ultrasound. Dr. Greenberg served as medical advisor to the Florida Department of Professional Regulation, Board of Medicine. He has also served as a member of the board of trustees of the HCA Medical Center of Port St. Lucie. He currently is Associate Professor of Medicine, Division of Rheumatology, University of South Carolina School of Medicine.

Nathan Wei, MD, FACP, FACR is a graduate of Swarthmore College and the Jefferson Medical College. He completed his residency at the University of Michigan Medical Center in Ann Arbor, Michigan and his fellowship in arthritis at the National Institutes of Health in Bethesda, Maryland. Dr. Wei is an acknowledged national expert in rheumatoid arthritis and osteoarthritis and is the author of more than 500 publications.

He is a Fellow of the American College of Physicians, a Fellow of the American College of Rheumatology, and is the only American rheumatologist member in the Arthroscopy Association of North America. He is considered an authority and expert in stem cell and platelet-rich plasma (PRP) procedures. He is active in clinical research and is the Director of the Arthritis Treatment Center, located in Frederick, Maryland.

INTRODUCTION
What This book Is All About

Let's begin, nor with the beginning, but with the moment a patient enters our office. The actual beginning, as far as the patient is concerned, was when the symptoms first appeared. Unfortunately, as we will see, many patients may wait weeks, months, or even years before they consult their doctor.

> Does your story resemble any one of the following?

> *Doctor, I can't deal with this pain in my hands any more. 1 thought I could live with it, but now I can scarcely put on my blouse, let alone manage by myself.*

The most many people hope for is a way to cope with chronic pain. Only when the pain becomes intolerable will they see their doctor.

> *The stiffness in my neck is terrible in the* morning. *I can't move my head; even my shoulders ache. It always goes away by afternoon, though.*

More often than not, victims of pain manage to get by, developing lifestyles to accommodate their suffering. Perhaps a general practitioner years ago prescribed aspirin for the treatment of their symptoms, and they haven't seen a doctor about the problem since. They feel that they already know what the physician is going to say, so why waste the money?

> *But the doctor said it was arthritis!*

These arc just some of the stories we hear from our patients every day at our medical offices. As rheumatologists, we advertise ourselves as "arthritis specialists,"—doctors with knowledge and insight about pain in the bones, joints, and muscles—so it makes sense that the patients we most often see are those who sincerely believe that they have arthritis.

Quite apart from the pain and physical discomfort that goes with the condition, arthritis seems to give rise to a particular mindset about suffering: that arthritis is chronic and incurable. The moment the mere notion of it enters the picture, many people abandon all hope for a normal, active day-to-day life. And once they accept chronic pain as permanent, they become oddly willing to put up with it and develop lifestyles geared toward coping with their suffering. The result is often they will not see a regular doctor—let alone a specialist—until they cannot deal with the pain any longer.

No one should have to live with such suffering. And yet, the chances are that if you are browsing in this book, say, in the health section of your local bookstore or library, you are probably suffering a great deal from persistent pain in your back or your neck—enough, certainly, to want to do something about it.

The chances are also pretty good that you believe you have arthritis. What is arthritis? Arthritis is rather like pornography: people can't define it but they know it when they feel it. Arthritis simply means "joint inflammation," and what it describes is not so much a specific disease as a condition, a symptom that can result from any one of over 100 causes, ranging from viral and bacterial infection to bad nutrition, to the side-effects of certain medications. The sad irony is that many of the problems people call "arthritis"—that incurable, inevitable scourge of old age—are very often afflictions that are highly treatable, even curable, by conventional medicine.

This is the good news we have to offer—with the right treatment, you may find an end finally to your suffering. The problem for doctors and patients alike is how to arrive at the proper diagnosis. As you will see, so many different conditions can lead to the same problem. That swollen knee or a burning sensation in the foot may be caused by a dozen different diseases. It's no wonder that confusion reigns: self-diagnosis, misdiagnosis, and no diagnosis are all too often the rule of the day, leading not only to inadequate treatment, but sometimes to inappropriate, even harmful treatment. A doctor cannot identify an ailment properly without the right information, and a patient cannot be expected to know in advance what information the doctor will need to diagnose properly.

Doctor, Why Do I Hurt So Much! is first and foremost an attempt to create a partnership between you and your doctor, with the goal of providing you substantive relief from your suffering. By "substantive relief," we mean treatment that addresses not only symptoms, but causes as well—treatment that enables you to enjoy a healthier, happier life.

In this book, we present a three-stage program to teach you how to help your doctor arrive at appropriate diagnoses for your ailments:

    1) Where does it hurt?
    2) How does it hurt? and
    3) What can I do?

First, by learning to identify the nature and location of your pain, then by learning how to recount your medical history, you will enable the doctor to gather the information needed to make a sound determination as to the cause of the affliction. Only when this has been done will the doctor be able to prescribe an effective treatment plan that should alleviate your needless suffering.

In that sense, one might think of Doctor, Why *Do I Hurt So* Much? is a kind of anti-arthritis book. By placing arthritis in the greater context of the musculoskeletal system, we believe that we will be able to alleviate much of the fear and anxiety surrounding arthritis and inspire you to seek competent medical advice.

Take as an example chronic stiffness in the neck. A stiff neck feels like arthritis, but it may be the result of *osteoarthritis,* the common "wear-and-tear" arthritis, *fibromyalgia,* in which the patient experiences increased muscle tension in the neck associated with exquisitely sensitive trigger points as well as fatigue, depression, and poor quality sleep, or *ankylosing spondylitis,* in which the bones in the neck fuse together, restricting one's ability to turn the head or look up and down.

To complicate matters further, people often confuse symptoms. Some people may verbalize that they have "neck pain" when they really have muscle weakness or stiffness. Thus, the patient's "arthritic neck pain" may actually be the result of such different afflictions as *myositis* or *polymyalgia rheumatica.*

Finally, the problem the patient is having in the neck may not be the direct result of any disease or injury. Rather, it may be the side effect of a medication, the outcome of a vitamin deficiency, or the result of over accumulation of minerals in the body. In other words, what people often call "arthritis" may not even be arthritis at all.

The complexity of issues surrounding the musculoskeletal system is such that the individual must learn to recognize and identify any number of symptoms above and beyond the stiff neck or the swollen knee.

Before we can begin to treat your ailment, we—both you the patient and we the physicians—have to give up the idea that we already know what it is and what is causing it. In this book, you will see the first requirement for arriving at the proper treatment for your affliction is for you to avoid the pitfalls of self-diagnosis. As any good doctor will tell you, it is far better to ask the right questions than to know all the answers.

First, an overview of *Doctor, Why Do I Hurt So Much?*
Part 1: Where does it hurt?

All too often in medical treatment, assumptions are made about physical conditions without adequate information. In Part One, we will teach you how to develop an overview of your condition. We will introduce you to the idea of a *pain journal,* in which you will learn how to keep a diary of the manifestations of your ailment, beginning with the identification of the location and the nature of your complaint. When do you feel bad? Where do you feel your pain? Equally important, when and how do you obtain comfort and relief? Only after learning how to document your current problem and also your personal medical history can you help your doctor sort relevant from irrelevant data in determining the diagnosis.

Part 2: How does it hurt?

As we noted in the example of the chronically stiff neck, a single problem may he indicative of any one of a number of different afflictions. In Part Two, we explore how pain affects different parts of the body and examine the different causes that might lead to that pain. Because many musculoskeletal conditions are so often confused with arthritis, we begin with a discussion of arthritis and the general types of disease associated with it, most notably the CORE diseases (Crystal diseases, Osteoarthritis, Rheumatoid arthritis & Connective Tissue Diseases, Enthesopathies). We also examine fatigue, muscle pain and weakness as well as a variety of diseases that have musculoskeletal symptoms.

With these discussions as a foundation, we then examine how pain manifests itself in different parts of the body and its possible causes.

While Part One and the opening chapters of Part Two will contain information pertinent to every reader's situation, the subsequent chapters on diagnosis are self-contained. That is, if you are experiencing sensitivity in the upper arm and shoulder, you can turn directly to the sections on those parts of the body.

Part 3: What can I do?

The underlying purpose of *Doctor, Why Do I Hurt So Much?* is to provide you the wherewithal to help your doctor make the best possible diagnosis of the cause of your suffering. As such, it is not so much a self-help book as a book designed to help you understand the kind of information the doctor needs to be able to provide sound, practical treatment.

In Part Three, we look at various "lifestyle" issues and how they might contribute to your condition. From nutrition and dietary supplements to the side effects of drugs and medications, we examine how what we take in affects the body. Of special interest are comprehensive tables listing vitamins, minerals, food types, and drugs along with their various side-effects.

The last chapter, "Regaining Control," presents advice on how to find the right doctor. While all doctors are licensed in the states where they practice, the profusion of specialists makes it difficult to know what kind of doctor you should approach for the treatment of your affliction. Moreover, as we become increasingly mobile, the ideal of the hometown doctor who's known you all your life is becoming more and more impossible to realize.

In regaining control, while you are seeking help for your affliction, you are also seeking to establish a partnership with your doctor, a relationship in which both sides are equal. What do you need to know about your doctor to make the right choice?

Developing a partnership with your physician

What we are proposing is a three-stage program to help you learn the answer to two questions: Why are you in pain? And, more importantly, what can you do about it? A correct diagnosis is based upon good information. We encourage you to take an active role in determining the cause of your pain by teaching you to communicate key information to your doctor. Despite all the technological advances in medicine made in recent years, the single most useful tool that a physician has in identifying disease remains the patient history, your account of your medical background. Your history, your *story* will provide your physician the most important clues he or she will need in the investigation of your problem. Only when the doctor understands the exact source of your pain can he or she develop the most appropriate treatment.

This book is *not* designed to help you arrive at some form of self-diagnosis.

Interpreting medical information and forming a correct diagnosis is the job of the physician. Nor is this hook encyclopedic in the sense that it covers all possible causes for all possible pains. Finally, it cannot take the place of the physical examination and the variety of tests available.

Doctor, Why Do I Hurt So Much? is, essentially another diagnostic tool—one that we hope will give you the means of participating in the treatment, if not the actual cure, of your affliction. Arthritis is *not a glamorous disease.*

Ironically, nothing we will tell you in this book is particularly new, though in the interest of our patients, our practice, and in the columns we write for various publications, we do keep up with the latest research on the musculoskeletal system. Indeed, it is a terribly sad thing that although we are well into the 21th century, there are still many people who suffer from "arthritic" diseases that have been treatable for years.

Part of the dilemma, no doubt, has to do with the changing nature of modern medicine. Somewhere between the eye-catching dramatic diseases that appeal to the media, and our society's relentless drive for longevity, we *all* lose sight of the problem of chronic pain. There are few arthritis-sufferer support groups; there is no arthritis hotline. Indeed, many doctors have no formal training in either arthritis or the type of chronic pain associated with the condition because most teaching hospitals concentrate on acute illness and severe, life-threatening medical problems. Few offer courses on such mundane problems as the painful shoulder or the swollen knee.

But as we have learned over our years of practice, pain, especially chronic pain, erodes the *quality of life.* So much of what we encounter in our office is the combination *of* fear, stress, anxiety, and depression that often follows just this kind of suffering. While a thorough and individual evaluation of the patient's condition may simply bring some peace of mind, the fact remains that to treat a patient properly, the physician must attend to the entire patient, and not just to the back or the knee.

As we have also learned, completeness, this regard for the patient's entire *being* has its own, and often not too predictable, rewards. Rather like detectives, we find that the overlooked clue in the medical history, the seemingly unrelated problem in another part of the body, the curious reaction to a particular kind of food—these all may shed enormous light on the main problem. And that, in its turn, will lead us to prescribe an appropriate treatment plan.

How to use this book

Now that you know our grand scheme and the overall outline of the book, you can put our work to use. Chapters 1 through 4 and chapter 12 are intended for every reader. As you learn first to identity the nature and location of your pain, then the ways you experience and alleviate it, and finally how to recount your medical history, you should then understand your problem well enough to consider it within the overall context of arthritis.

For many, the core of this book will be chapter 5, "Parts of the Body Affected." Organized by body area, this chapter allows you to explore the various ailments that *might*—and we emphasize the word *might*—be contributing to your condition. In this chapter, you need only turn to those portions that pertain to the parts of the body where you are experiencing pain. Rather than giving you fixed answers, our purpose here is to alert you to the possible causes and describe in very broad terms the variety of treatments that can be prescribed.

While we described this earlier as an *anti-arthritis* book, many readers may well believe that they are suffering from arthritis of some kind. Thus, in chapter 6, we describe the major arthritis groups. We are not asking you at this point to determine whether or not you have arthritis; rather, we are simply laying the facts on the table for your consideration.

Similarly, chapters 7 through 9 recount other diseases and afflictions that cause the kind of musculoskeletal pain that is often confused with arthritis. Again, we ask you to withhold drawing any conclusions about your particular condition.

Thus prepared, you will be able to enter a meaningful partnership with your physician. Then and only then will you undergo the examination and tests needed to arrive at a proper diagnosis and set you on your way to an appropriate treatment plan.

In chapters 10 and 11, we examine the most common outside agents that may be contributing to your condition. Again, these two chapters—the first pertaining to nutrition and dietary supplements, the second to drugs and their side-effects—are not intended to give you ready answers to your complaints. Unfortunately, there has been very little research into the relationship between diet and pain, and there probably will not be until the medical establishment acknowledges the role of diet in our daily lives. Look up the foods and supplements you eat both regularly and on occasion and see if they might be contributing to your condition.

As for chapter 11, dealing with the side effects of drugs and medications, the research is ongoing. And while pharmaceutical companies and physicians attempt to arrive at a complete picture of how drugs and medications work prior to their release on the general population, the fact remains that many of these "products" might affect our bodies in ways that lab and test trials cannot anticipate. So, as with the chapter on diet and dietary supplements, these tables are far from being either complete or conclusive.

Lastly, in chapter 12, "Regaining Control," we offer advice on how to find the right doctor with whom to pursue your diagnosis and treatment. In this era of proliferating specialties, the endless panoply of internists, cardiologists, this-ists and that-ists is daunting.

Our hope is that with these suggestions you will encounter a physician who will enable you to regain a better quality of life.

PART ONE:
WHERE DOES IT HURT?

When is it that what we feel is not *well*? Typically, we associate well-being with normality, but all too often for all too many people, normality involves measures of discomfort and dysfunction.

Does this describe your situation? Have you lost sight of the difference between what you *can* and what you *should* be able to do? Have you denied the experience of your physical pain, gradually restricting your activities and your sense of independence to accommodate your suffering?

What we are discussing here is *chronic pain* and not the temporary discomfort which is generally nothing to worry about. *Chronic pain* is persistent, disruptive, and restrictive. It occurs regularly. It disrupts your day-to-day activities. It restricts your ability to move, to take care of yourself, to be independent.

Chronic, persistent pain may be an indication of a significant problem or a more generalized disease. And because pain can originate from a variety of sources—nerves, bone, or other tissue— diagnosing pain is no simple task. But it is something you must be able to do if you want to describe your condition to your doctor accurately.

How Pain is Diagnosed

A physician generally examines pain from three fronts: medical history, physical examination, and diagnostic tests.

Your medical history will be discussed in greater detail in chapter 3. In the physical examination, the physician observes, listens, pokes, prods, presses, and taps in order to find clues both obvious and subtle regarding your condition. The third front upon undiagnosed pain is the laboratory test and X-rays, as well as such technological wonders as musculoskeletal ultrasound, magnetic resonance imaging and electrophysiological studies of nerves and muscles. Although such testing is becoming increasingly sophisticated, the results must be seen within the framework of the patient's overall condition.

From these three sources, the physician must find reasonable compatibility among the history, the physical examination, and the lab results to arrive at an appropriate diagnosis. A diagnosis that disregards evidence from all three sources—the history, the physical exam, and the lab work—is the one most likely to be misleading. The question is how to sort through the data to arrive at a good diagnosis.

For example, many patients with *lupus erythematosus* (an inflammatory connective tissue disease) will have a falsely positive test for syphilis. However, because the history and physical examination of patients with these diseases are generally so different, it is very rare that a physician will confuse the two.

What further complicates arriving at a diagnosis is that diseases can, and frequently do, occur in combination. Having *rheumatoid arthritis* or *lupus* does not grant you immunity from developing *osteoarthritis, gout,* or any other such problem. For example, if your condition disrupts your sleep, part of your aching may *be fibromyalgia,* in which exquisitely painful trigger points develop in your soft tissues.

Along with the three-point approach to the diagnosis of pain, then we must add a fourth: your own description of the kind of pain you feel. *Where* do you feel it? *How* you feel it? *When* you feel it?

Structures of Pain

Pain may have its origins in bone, nerves, body organs, and/ or soft tissues, all of which we discuss in chapter 5, "Parts of the Body Affected." As living matter, these structures can be affected by physical injury, infection, and disease, all of which can result in pain. But when an individual says, "Ow! It hurts!", the pain can be manifesting in a variety of ways, each of which feels distinctly different.

What follows are general rules of thumb to help you describe your pain.

Is It Hot or Not?

Distinguishing between non-inflammatory and inflammatory types of pain is very important for diagnostic purposes. However, inflammation may be very difficult even for an experienced specialist to detect.

Inflamed joints classically are red, hot, swollen, and tender, but these symptoms often occur only in matters of degree. The most telling sign of inflammation is a sense of stiffness in the joint or muscle, particularly after resting. This is called the "gelling phenomenon," and is rather like what happens to gelatin after it has been placed in the refrigerator. As it cools, gelatin solidifies and stiffens. When it is taken out of the refrigerator, it takes a while to achieve room temperature, when it begins to liquefy or loosen up.

This is what happens in the joints and muscles of a patient who has an inflammatory disease: As the patient rests, the joints and muscles stiffen. If a joint or muscle is stiff for more than an hour after resting, most physicians agree it is a sign of significant inflammation.

Other Types of Pain Sensation:
Expanding Your Vocabulary For Pain

Each person feels pain in his or her own way. So the general ways pain is described may differ dramatically. However, most people agree that a *stabbing pain* is very much like having a knife stuck in them. *Pressure* causes the sensation of being squeezed. *Locking in* feels as if the joint cannot be moved, and when it does, it has a distinctive popping as it is set into motion.

Similarly, there is *burning* (often associated with inflammation), tingling ("pins and needles"), and *stiffness* or *tightness.*

Whatever words you use, though, describe the pain naturally. Can you visualize it? Is it cold or hot? Is it tender or numb? The better you put it into words, the better your physician will be able to arrive at a good diagnosis.

Now that you've learned some of the ways in which we identify pain, let's look at one of the most effective tools the patient has to offer the physician, the *pain journal.*

If the notion of dwelling on your suffering somehow is abhorrent to you, remember that this is an important step in getting sound treatment. The better able you are to describe the nature of your pain, the better informed your doctor will be to arrive at an appropriate diagnosis. It really is that simple.

Your doctor will want to know three basic things about your pain: *Where? How? When?* The "where" refers to the part or parts of the body affected—not just the feet or the arms, but the precise location of the pain. The "how" refers to the kind of pain you feel as discussed in chapter 1.

"When" is perhaps the most difficult question to answer of the three. If you have been living with chronic pain, the chances are very good that you have begun to feel that it is constant. But in this exercise, you will have to pay particular attention to your pain. When does it feel worse? When does it feel better? What do you do to alleviate your pain? If you have been living with this condition long enough, you may very well be unaware of how you have been treating your ailment.

Where?

In the main, it is easiest to say "where" it hurts—the shoulder, for example, or the knee. The problem comes in learning to be as specific as possible. The next time you feel discomfort, try to be conscious of the precise location of the pain.

Say you are having trouble with your elbow. Does the pain seem to come from the center of the joint or do you feel it particularly on one side or the other?

What if the pain is in your hands? As you will see in the chapter on parts of the body affected, different locations of pain in the hand can signify very different ailments. Do you feel the pain most acutely in your little finger or does it come from the middle or index finger? The same goes for your feet. Pinpoint where you feel the pain most.

There are times when pain is not so localized. You may feel pain all along the inside of your forearm or all along the back of your lower leg. This is especially true for certain kinds of physical injury in which the muscle or tendon has been aggravated by overuse or improper stress.

None of this is to suggest that you should only feel pain in one place. Some diseases attack different places at once. *Carpal tunnel syndrome* affects the wrist and hand but may also affect the forearm. *Fibromyalgia* causes numerous trigger points of pain in the soft-tissue areas of the body. These can appear in the upper back, the thigh, the arms, and the neck—anywhere where there is muscle mass. Sometimes, though, the question of "where" is complicated by the fact that certain pains seem to "travel." That is, you might be experiencing pain at different times in different parts of the body.

As you try to chronicle the "where" of your pain, bear in mind that there are no wrong answers. Whether you are feeling pain in only one place or in various parts of your body—beneath your kneecap or all over your upper torso—the purpose here is to give as precise and complete a description of where you hurt as possible.

Figure 1 on the next page is a body illustration provided for your convenience. It may be useful for you to shade in the areas of your discomfort for reference. In chapter 5, "Parts of the Body Affected" you can use your own "pain diagram" to help you and your doctor define your problem.

How?

We have already touched upon this a bit in the previous chapter by introducing you to a vocabulary of pain. Inflammation— when the affected area is typically hot, swollen, and tender to the touch—is a very particular kind of pain, though it can signify different causes, depending on its location. An inflamed joint or muscle is different from an inflamed appendix.

Do you feel stiff after resting? Does it take real effort to get the joint or muscle moving? Or is the stiffness constant—that is, does it feel as if it never really goes away?

Are you experiencing a *stabbing pain?* Or does it feel as if the affected area is being squeezed? If it is occurring in a joint, does it feel as if your bones have somehow become locked together?

At times, "how" is rather like "where": a *travelling pain* seems to start in one place and go to another, like a telegraph. And there are types of pain that simply seem to make you hurt "all over."

When?

 Like a detective in a mystery, a physician needs to know not just the "where" and the "how" but the "when" of your pain as well.

Burning, tingling, tight, raw, deep, superficial, passing, constant, spinning, nauseous: these are some very useful words in describing how it hurts. In the case of suffering, "when" refers actually to two different periods of time: when you first felt the pain, and when you feel the pain in your day-to-day living.

When you first began to feel this pain—it may have been recently or a long time ago—perhaps you were thinking that it might simply go away. (How many times have we heard that "time is the great healer"?) Perhaps it did, but now it has come back.

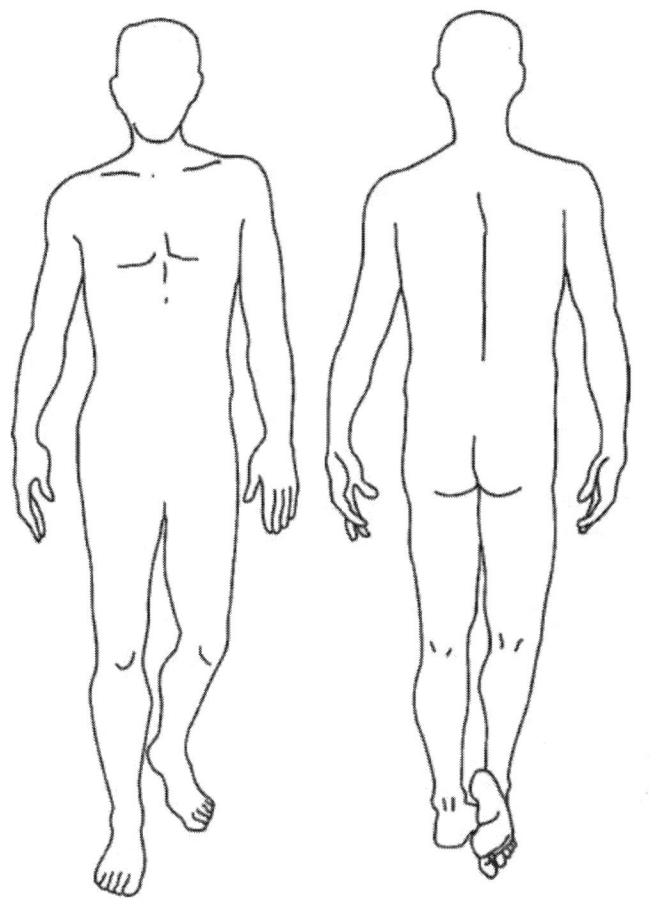

Figure 1- Your personal pain diagram.

So, the first part of "when" had to do with the chronology of your pain. When did it start? When did it go away? When did it come back? Some diseases work as regularly as clockwork, coming and going and coming again, so it's important to remember when they have affected you.

The second aspect of "when" is how you feel pain in your day-to-day life. Does it feel worse in the morning or at the end of the day? Do you feel it particularly when you have been doing a certain task, like sitting down or leaning over a counter or walking upstairs?

No less important than when it hurts is when it feels better. There may be some things you do that alleviate the pain. If you experience pain sitting down, for example, you may feel better when you stand up and walk around for a while. Maybe all you need to do is put your feet up and the pain goes away.

Whatever happens, your doctor needs to know when you hurt, when you feel better, and what you do that either makes you hurt or helps the pain go away.

Your Pain Journal

Now that you know the three basic questions, the next question is how to keep a record of your pain. How long should you do it? What kind of format should you follow?

There are no particular guidelines we think you should follow in writing up your pain journal. The important thing about the pain journal is that it can help you remember how the pain affects you and how it has affected your life. It does not have to be a meticulous diary kept day in and day out for years. What your doctor will want is some kind of idea of how the illness, as it has been manifested in your pain, has progressed over a certain period of time, whether it is only a week or whether it is three months.

This is particularly true if you have been suffering from chronic pain. As you begin to do your pain journal, you may be surprised at all the things you have forgotten about or overlooked. Chronic pain has a way of making you forget everything but the pain itself.

And that's why you are now going to see the doctor.

Chapter Three – *Recording Your Medical History*

No less important than the pain journal in the identification of disease is a complete and detailed account of your medical history. All too often, you are expected to fill in forms upon first arriving at the doctor's office. The result is that the record of your medical history is frequently rushed and sometimes quite confused.

Seemingly trivial and insignificant information can be overlooked and forgotten, while it might very well be that the original cause for the current problem lies in that shoulder that was broken way back when or in the side-effects of a medication that you no longer take.

For this reason, we encourage you to take a long and serious look at your own medical history. We also recommend that you try to record medical issues involving blood relatives. Is there a particular condition that occurs among various members of the family?

Lastly, where a somewhat impersonal "intake" interview might leave you too embarrassed to acknowledge how lifestyle affects well-being, such issues may be critical to understanding your present affliction. We allow the patient the privacy of completing the medical history in his or her own good time, with the hope that he or she will provide the most complete history possible.

What follows is an example of a medical history questionnaire. If you have had any experience with these, you will see that this is somewhat more detailed than most. Some of it you may find embarrassing; some of it you may find annoying. However, the more complete your responses, the better able the physician will be to develop a good overall understanding not only of your state of health, but also of the particular condition that is troubling you.

In preparation for a visit to your physician, you might want to make photocopies of this chapter. After all, it is easier to write on a flat sheet of paper than it is to write in a book.

Part 1. Past Medical History

1. List *all* prior medical problems, including cancer (type and location), stroke, heart attack, heart disease, diabetes, high blood pressure, anemia (low blood count), rheumatic fever, tuberculosis, thyroid disease (too fast or too slow), and gout. Also make reference to any prior diagnosis of arthritis and, if known, what form. Please give approximate dates of all prior ailments.

   _____

   _____

   _____

2. Please list any diseases that have affected *blood relatives*— parents, brothers, sisters, children, uncles, aunts, grandparents, and first cousins. Include diagnoses such as those listed above. Have any of your relatives had arthritis? Also indicate year of death where applicable.

   _____

   _____

3. List all medications you are currently taking, including ills, capsules, suppositories, injections, and patches. Also include over-the-counter medications, birth control pills, and vitamins. What dosage are you currently taking?

   Medication   Dose

   _____   ____ Per ____
   _____   ____ Per ____
   _____   ____ Per ____
   _____   ____ Per ____

   If you are taking more medications, please attach a separate sheet.

4. List all prior operations you have had (for example, tonsils and adenoids, gallbladder, appendectomy, hemorrhoids, joint replacements, Caesarian sections, neck or back operations, etc.) For each operation, list the year performed. If you have had a hysterectomy, include the reason for the operation and indicate whether the ovaries were removed or not.

_____

_____

_____

5. List all physical injuries and bone fractures (breaks) you have had. Indicate the parts of the body affected and the date of the injury.

_____

_____

_____

_____

6. List all Hospitalizations. Please list why, where, and when you were hospitalized.

_____

_____

_____

7. Women: Please list the number of children you have had and whether the child is living or dead. Where a child has died, please indicate the cause. In the case of miscarriages, indicate the approximate month of pregnancy during which it occurred.

_____

_____

_____

8. List any allergies and drug reactions that you have:

Medication *Allergy/Reaction*

_____ _____

_____ _____

_____ _____

_____ _____

9. Have you ever smoked cigarettes? ❑Yes ❑No
   Have you ever smoked cigars? ❑Yes ❑No

   If you answer yes to either question, indicate how long you have smoked and the number of cigarettes or cigars you smoke per day.

   _____

   _____

   _____

   If you have quit smoking, when did you stop? _____

10. Do you drink alcohol? ❑Yes ❑No
    Indicate the number of drinks (and type) you take on average in a week. Please include beer and wine.

    _____

    _____

    Have you ever used recreational drugs? ❑Yes ❑No
    If yes, which ones? _____

    _____

    Have you ever used intravenous drugs? ❑Yes ❑No
    Have you ever shared needles? ❑Yes ❑No

11. Please describe your sexual preference:

    _____

    _____

    Has this varied since adolescence? ❑Yes ❑No

12. Have you had more than one sexual partner in the past year?

_____

_____

13. Have you had any pets in the past ten years?

              ❑Yes ❑No

What kind of animal or animals? For cats, indicate whether the cat was a house cat or one that you allowed outside the house. Please list the dates:

_____

_____

14. Where have you traveled in the past ten years?

              ❑Yes ❑No

The U.S. Year   *Outside the U.S. Year*

_____

_____

_____

_____

15. Where have you lived over the past ten years? Please list where you have lived during that time and when:

_____

_____

_____

_____

16. Please list your occupations since you first entered the job market, including what you are currently doing.

_____

_____

_____

_____

17. Do you have any hobbies?   ❑Yes ❑No

_____
_____
_____
_____

18. Does either your work or your hobbies expose you to any chemicals?　　　　　　　　　❑Yes ❑No

If so, do you know what they are?

_____
_____
_____
_____

Part 2. Your Current Condition

What follows has been developed for the book. It includes much of the information that you would include in your pain journal

1. If you are experiencing a number of different pains, describe each one on a separate copy of this form.
   Pain
   location: _____

   _____

2. How severe is the pain? Use a scale of 0-10, with 10 being the most severe pain you have ever suffered.

   _____
   _____

3. How long has this area hurt you?
   a. Days: _____
   b. Weeks: _____
   c. Months: _____
   d. Years:_____

4. Is the pain constant or intermittent?   ❏Yes ❏No

   If intermittent, how long do the painful spells last?

   _____

   If constant, does the intensity of pain vary at times?

   _____

5. What activities aggravate or bring on the pain?

   _____

   _____

6. What activities alleviate or stop the pain?

   _____

   _____

7. Did the pain start suddenly or did it come on gradually?
                                            ❏Yes ❏No
   a. If suddenly, do you remember what you were doing when
      it occurred?

      _____

   b. If the onset was gradual, how long has it taken to develop?

      _____

8. How would you characterize the pain (sharp, achy, crampy, stiff,
   burning, shooting, stabbing, etc.)?

   _____

   _____

9. What treatments (medication, physical therapy, etc.) have been
   tried so far?

   _____

   Has any treatment
   helped? _____

   _____

   _____

10. Has the pain improved or worsened with time?

_____

11. Does the pain move anywhere?   ❑Yes ❑No

_____

12. Are there any other problems that seem to coincide with the pain? (For example, shortness of breath, a rash, chest pain, or fever)

_____

_____

13. If you are experiencing stiffness with this pain, how long does it last after waking up in the morning?
   a. Minutes _____
   b. Hours_____
   c. All day_____

If the pain is located in a joint or limb, do you notice any swelling where it hurts?

_____

_____

If a joint is involved, is movement difficult? Do you feel it locking (that is, does the joint "catch" when you straighten or bend it)?

_____

_____

Part 3. Overview of Your Medical Systems

1. Do you have fevers?   ❑Yes ❑No
    How high? _____

    Are they intermittent or constant? ❑intermittent ❑constant

2. If intermittent, how often do you have fevers?

_____

3. Do you experience sweats, chills, or both?

_____

If so, what time of day do they occur? _____

4. Have you noticed you have gained or lost weight recently?

❑ Gained   ❑ Lost   ❑No change

    a. If so, how much? _____ Pounds.
    b. Over how long a time did this weight change take place?

_____

_____

_____

5. Did you purposely try to gain or lose weight?_____

6. Do you feel weak?   ❑Yes ❑No
   Always or sometimes?   ❑Yes ❑No
   Do you feel it throughout your body or only in particular areas?
   What area(s)?

_____

7. Do you feel tired when you don't think you should be?
    a. ❑Yes ❑No
    b. Always or sometimes?   _____
    c. Is the fatigue severe or mild? _____
    d. For how long have you been aware of this? _____

_____

    e. Weeks _____
    f. Months _____
    g. Years _____

8. Do your muscles hurt?
   Which ones?
   Upper arms _____   Neck _____
   Calve_____   Thighs _____

Shoulder _____   Other _____

How would you describe the pain?
Cramping? _____
Aching? _____
Stiff?_____
Burning?_____
Other? _____

9. Do you sleep well at night?   ❑Yes ❑No
   If not, why not? _____
   Is it the result of pain? _____
   Does your mind "race"? _____
   Is there any other reason? _____
   Is this a recent problem?_____
   Do you usually wake up refreshed? _____

10. Do you have any swollen glands?   ❑Yes ❑No
    Where? _____
    For how long? _____

11. Have you had any skin rashes?   ❑Yes ❑No
    If so, where? _____

12. Do you often get mouth sores?   ❑Yes ❑No
    If so, how often? _____
    Are they painful? _____

13. Does your scalp hurt when you comb your hair?
                                         ❑Yes ❑No
    Have you experienced hair loss? _____
    If so, is it patchy or is the entire scalp involved? _____
    Over what period of time?_____

14. Do you have any skin ulcers, lumps, bumps, tightening?
    If so, where?_____

15. Do you have psoriasis (a certain skin disease):

    ❑Yes ❑No

16. In a cold environment (cold weather, for example, or the frozen foods section of supermarket), do your fingers feel very cold?

    ❑Yes ❑No

    Do they change color? ❑Yes ❑No

    If so, what colors do they become?

    _____

    _____

17. Have you noticed any changes in your fingernails?

    ❑Yes ❑No

    Are there tiny pits? ❑Yes ❑No

    Do the fingernails crack easily? ❑Yes ❑No

    Any other problem? ❑Yes ❑No

    _____

    _____

18. Do you get a rash in the sun? ❑Yes ❑No

    If so, what color is it? _____

    Does it itch? _____

    Where is it located? _____

19. Do you have frequent headaches? ❑Yes ❑No

    How often do they occur? _____

    Do you experience nausea with them? ❑Yes ❑No

    Do they affect your vision? _____ ❑Yes ❑No

    How? _____

    Are these headaches severe? ❑Yes ❑No

    When do you experience them? _____

    What relieves them? _____

    Where are the headaches located exactly? _

    _____

    _____

Have you ever been told that you have migraine headaches?

_____

_____

When did these headaches start?

_____

_____

20. Do you suffer from neck pain frequently? ❏Yes ❏No
Have you ever suffered an injury to your neck?

_____

_____

If so, how and when?

_____

_____

21. Have you noticed any problem with your hearing?

_____

_____

For how long? _____

_____

Is the problem in one ear or both? _____
Do you feel ear pain? _____
Do you have any ear discharge? _____

22. Do you have dry eyes or dry mouth often? (circle which)
Do you feel that your eyes water excessively?

_____

23. Have you ever had conjunctivitis or any other form of eye
inflammation?

_____

_____

If so, what did you have and
when? _____

_____

Were you given cortisone eye drops? _____

24. Do you have frequent nosebleeds, sore throat, sinus problems, post-nasal drip? _____

_____

25. Do you have pain in your jaw when you chew?

_____

_____

Does your tongue hurt when you talk? __❑Yes ❑No

26. Do you have chest pain?   ❑Yes ❑No
    If so, where?_____
    Does it move? _____
    Does it change when you take a deep breath?

    _____

    Does your body position affect the pain in any way?

    _____

    Is the pain associated with shortness of breath, nausea, vomiting, or excessive sweating?

    _____

    What brings it on?

    _____

    _____

    ❑ Exertion?   ❑ Eating too much?
    ❑ Cold weather?   ❑ Stress?
    ❑ What alleviates the pain?   ❑ Rest?
    ❑ Antacid?   ❑ Other? _____

27. Do you have a cough?   ❑Yes ❑No
    Does it produce sputum or phlegm?   If so, what color?

    _____

    Is this a new occurrence or is it chronic?

    _____

Does it occur only when you are lying flat in bed?

_____

28. Are you often short of breath? _____
    If so, does lying flat aggravate it? _____
    Does it occur with exertion? _____
    If so, how many blocks do you walk before you feel short of breath?

    _____

    How many stairs can you climb before you feel short of breath?

    _____

    Have you ever experienced any wheezing? _____
    Asthma? _____
    Episodes of bronchitis? _____ Pneumonia? _____
    Pleurisy? _____
    If you have experienced any of the above, how frequently do you
    suffer from such respiratory disorders?

    _____

    _____

29. Have you ever experienced palpitations or the sensation that
    your heart is "thumping" or "racing" in your chest?
    If so, how often does this occur?_____
    Have you ever had heart rhythm problems?

    _____

    _____

    Have you ever had heart failure?

    _____

    _____

    Do you have a heart murmur?

    _____

    _____

30. Have you ever experienced swelling in the lower leg?

    _____

    _____

    Does this occur at a particular time of day? _____

    _____

Are your legs entirely normal in the morning? _____

_____

31. Do you frequently experience nausea or vomiting? How is your appetite?
Poor? _____
Fair? _____
"Too Good"? _____
Do you have any difficulty swallowing? If so, do you have trouble with:
Solid foods? _____
Liquids? _____
Both? _____
For how long has swallowing been a problem? _____

_____
Have you ever had any ulcers? _____
In the stomach? _____
In the duodenum? _____
Did the ulcer bleed? _____

32. Have you ever had hepatitis or yellow jaundice?
❏Yes ❏No
If so, when did this occur? _____
What type of hepatitis was it? _____
Have you ever had a dark or bloody stool?
❏Yes ❏No
Do you ever find bright red blood on the toilet paper or on your stool? _____
Do you experience chronic constipation or diarrhea?
Which? _____
Do they occur together at times? _____
In general, are your bowel movements regular?
❏Yes ❏No
How often do you have a bowel movement?

_____

_____
Is the stool solid? _____

Do you notice any fatty or greasy particles in your stool ?

❏Yes ❏No

Have you noticed any change in your bowel habits?

❏Yes ❏No

If so, what is the change? _____

33. Do you have to wake up at night to urinate? _____

If so, how often? _____

Do you urinate frequently during the day? _____

If so, how often? _____

Do you have pain when you urinate? _____

Do you lose urine sometimes? _____

Does loss of urine occur only when you cough, sneeze, or laugh?

_____

Do you notice any blood in the urine?_____

Males: Has the force of the urine stream decreased?

Have you had difficulty in starting to urinate? _____

Females Have you had frequent urinary tract infections?

_____

Do you have significant vaginal discharge? _____

Have you ever had a venereal or sexually transmitted disease?

_____

_____

34. *Females:* Have you had any spotting between your menstrual periods? _____

When did you start having menstrual periods? _____

When did you stop? _____

If applicable, what form of contraception do you use?

Have you ever been pregnant? _____

Have you ever had a miscarriage or an abortion? _____

If so, how many? _____

In which month of pregnancy did this occur? _____

35. Males: Have you ever had difficulty in obtaining an erection? If so, for how long has this been a problem? _____

_____

Have you ever had this problem evaluated? _____

Have you ever had a prostate infection? _____

Have you ever had discharge from the penis? _____

Has anyone ever diagnosed urethritis? _____

Have you ever had a venereal or sexually transmitted disease?

_____

_____

36. Do you experience back pain or stiffness? _____

Have you ever had a back injury? _____

Is your back pain intermittent or constant? _____

What position or activity aggravates your back pain?

_____

What position alleviates your back pain? _____

_____

Is the pain severe? _____

Does the pain seem to move?

_____

_____

If it moves down the leg, which leg? _____

What part of the leg (outer or inner side, the front or the back?

_____

_____

How far down does the pain travel? _____

Does sitting down stop the pain? _____

Does lying in bed stop the pain? _____

Is the back pain accompanied by weakness or stiffness in the leg?

_____

_____

If walking brings on the back pain, how far must you walk before you feel the pain in your back? _____

_____

37. If we have not yet covered your problem, what joints hurt you?

_____

_____

Is there swelling associated with the joint pain?

_____

_____

In which joints? _____

Is there stiffness? _____

If so, how long does it last? _____

Is there any redness in and around the joint? _____

What aggravates the pain? _____

What alleviates the pain? _____

38. Do you have any dizziness? _____
Do you ever feel "woozy" or that you are "graying out"?

_____

_____

Do you ever had a spinning sensation?_____
If so for any of the above, how long? _____
Is it intermittent or chronic? _____
Does it occur when you stand up? _____
Does it occur when you lay your head back? _____
Have you experienced ringing in your ears? _____

Have you ever experienced a convulsion or seizure?

_____

_____

What were the circumstances? _____

Have you had any memory changes in the past few years?

_____

_____

Do you feel that this has been beyond "the normal aging process? _____

_____

Have you ever hit your head and passed out unconscious?

_____

Are you aware of any permanent damage? _____

_____

If so, what?

_____

_____

Did you simply pass out without hitting your head?

_____

What were the circumstances? _____

_____

Do your ears ring? _____
Intermittently or chronically? _____
Do you experience numbness, tingling, burning or
other unusual sensations? _____

_____

Do you feel this in your face? _____

If so, what part of the face is involved? _____

What brings on the pain and what stops it? _____

Do you feel similar pains in your hands? _____

The palm? _____ The fingers? _____
Which fingers? _____
Do you feel similar pain in your feet? _____
Which part of the foot? _____ Toes? _____
Which toes? _____

PART TWO:
HOW DOES IT HURT?

Chapter Four - *Do I Have Arthritis?*

Arthritis in its most basic sense simply means "joint inflammation." A joint is a place in the skeleton where two bones are connected in a way that allows movement.

Inflammation is just as it sounds: the joint swells, becomes hot, looks red, and is difficult to move.

While it is easy to recognize arthritis, many people probably do not realize that modern medicine has identified over 100 different types of arthritis—a number that continues to increase with our knowledge and awareness of the condition.

This is not to say that these are new types of arthritis—though with environmental change and our increasing exposure to un-known chemicals and hazardous waste, we cannot be entirely sure—but research has allowed us a deeper appreciation of the many factors that figure in the condition.

What if your joints hurt but are not necessarily inflamed? Or what if your muscles are causing you so much pain? In the first case, you'd have *arthralgia.* In the second case, you'd have *myalgia.* Arth- refers to the joint; *my-* or *myo-* means muscle; *algia* refers to pain. Just as arthritis only describes a particular condition—an inflamed joint *(itis* means literally "to set on fire")—arthralgia and myalgia merely say that you are experiencing pain in the joint or the muscle.

In a similar vein, *myositis* describes inflamed muscles—they become red, swollen, hot, stiff, tender, painful, and eventually weakened. With *myalgia,* though, the muscle simply hurts.

To put this all into plain English, you can have *arthralgia* (pain in your joints) without having *arthritis* (an inflamed joint), but you usually can't have arthritis without experiencing arthralgia as well. The same holds true for myositis and myalgia.

This isn't wordplay; these different classifications aren't just technicalities. They enable doctors to separate various types of joint and muscle pain into clearly defined groups. This, in turn, aids diagnosis. If we know specifically not only what joint or muscle is causing pain, but what kind of process is affecting the joint or muscle, it is much easier to formulate an appropriate diagnosis.

Thus the pain that people often call "arthritis" is not necessarily true arthritis. The following patient histories show how the precise definition of pain and its causes will dispel some common misconceptions about arthritis. These stories all have one thing in common: all of these patients came to our office believing that they had arthritis.

> *Susan, a 44-year-old executive secretary,* had been going from doctor to doctor to find the cause not only of her episodes of severe chest, back, and neck pain, but also of her constant fatigue. Over nearly a year, she had spent thousands of dollars on visits to general practitioners and specialists without experiencing significant improvement in her condition.
>
> By the time she came to us, she had begun to feel that her doctors were treating her like a hypochondriac. She was even beginning to think that perhaps they were right.
>
> After a session of detailed questioning, we discovered, among other things, that her dog had been waking her up at night. Her sleep disrupted, she had developed a soft tissue disease called *fibromyalgia*. This condition, in which the soft tissues develop deep aching, is often associated with the lack of good quality sleep. Moreover, she had developed numerous painful areas or "trigger points" in her back, neck, and chest.
>
> We had to do nothing in particular to treat her condition. Susan called her veterinarian, who prescribed a mild

sedative for her dog. After two nights of deep, sound sleep, Susan's pain disappeared and her energy returned.

Gertrude, a woman in her mid-fifties, described several weeks of intermittent severe tenderness in her joints and muscles. The joints sometimes became swollen and the swelling could last for several days. She recalled that before development of her condition, she had a red rash on her neck which improved slowly before disappearing. She was sure at first that it was arthritis.

But after reading a magazine article about *Lyme disease,* which is transmitted by a tick bite, Gertrude wondered if she might not have Lyme disease instead. She lived in an area where these ticks could be found, but she could not remember ever having been bitten. Sure enough, a blood test proved that her guess was right. It was positive for Lyme disease. A course of penicillin resulted in a complete cure.

John, a 71-year-old man, had been made miserable by an achy stiffness in his upper arms and shoulders that had been going on for the last three months. Though he had had pain on and off in his knees and hands for many years, this new pain seemed to be different. He had found it increasingly difficult to sleep and was exhausted during the day. To make matters worse, he had developed low back discomfort in the last month.

After questioning, examination, and a lab work-up, we found that John was experiencing three diseases. First off, he did in fact have arthritis—*osteoarthritis,* commonly known as "wear-and-tear arthritis"—in his hands and knees. The cartilage breaks down within the joint and the bones and the joints attempt to repair the damage by producing more bone.

The second problem we identified was the achy stiffness in his upper arms and shoulders. *Polymyalgia rheumatica (poly-* means multiple and *myalgia,* as we noted before, means muscle pain) had struck throughout his shoulders and upper arms. We treated this with a low-dose cortisone medication called prednisone, which completely relieved the pain in his shoulders and arms.

The sleeplessness provoked by the polymyalgia rheumatica pain had, in its turn, caused the trouble in John's lower back—the same *fibromyalgia* from which Susan was suffering. As the prednisone treatment began to take effect, John was able to sleep well, so his exhaustion disappeared and with it went his back pain.

Upon further examination, the osteoarthritis in his hands and knees did not seem to be severe, and John was able to control it, as he always had, with aspirin.

Bill, a 37-year-old executive, was referred to us by his general practitioner when treatment for the stiffness in his hands had proved ineffective, even after three months. The discomfort in his hands specifically involved the knuckles of his two fifth fingers.

One element of his medical history was particularly striking: his family had a history of diabetes. This raised the possibility that he himself was suffering from *hemochromatosis,* a genetic disease in which the body absorbs too much iron. With this disease, the excess iron enters not only into such organs as the liver, heart, and pancreas, but also into the joints, causing both *arthralgia* and *arthritis.*

The blood tests, which showed very high iron levels, reinforced the initial diagnosis and a liver biopsy confirmed it. Bill was treated with regular phlebotomy (a drawing off of blood), which lowered his body stores of iron. The stiffness in his fifth fingers gradually improved and the potential damage the excess iron might have done to his liver, heart, and pancreas was avoided.

The diabetes experienced by other members of his family was possibly caused by the infiltration of excess iron in the pancreas. Blood tests of all family members revealed several relatives who also had *hemochromatosis.* Happily, some of them had not yet suffered irreversible damage to the liver, heart, or pancreas, and like Bill, they were able to profit from the phlebotomy treatments.

What all of these examples show is that arthritis is not necessarily arthritis. Of course, while you might have osteoarthritis like John, you cannot be sure unless you have had a thorough medical examination. What feels like arthritis to you may actually be arthralgia or a symptom of a disease that may be far more dangerous than just a little stiffness in the joints. Perhaps it is an excess of foreign matter building up in the joints, as we discovered with Bill. Or it might very well be a low-grade inflammation of the soft tissues.

Whatever the case, there is a big difference between guessing you have arthritis and taking the time and effort to learn what it is that is working in your system. All of these patients— and many more— assumed they had arthritis. And while some were wrong, they were all concerned enough to see their doctors and persistent enough to find a physician who could sort through the data to arrive at a sound diagnosis which, in turn, led to their effective treatment.

Chapter Five – *Parts of the Body Affected*

Now as we begin to understand the variety of diseases that cause arthritis and other painful conditions, it's time to see how these and other diseases and ailments may be affecting you or someone close to you. The best place to begin the search for the cause of your discomfort is the specific part of the body where you are experiencing pain. Review your pain journal and read the sections of this chapter that might pertain to your particular problem. Afterwards, write down the possible causes and take the list with you when you see your doctor.

The diseases cited here may sound unfamiliar at first, so you might want to look over other chapters (especially chapters 6, 8, and 9) for specific descriptions of the diseases. To find the reference you want, simply check the index at the back of the book. Remember to look at the specific as well as the general picture to see if it pertains to your particular case.

Please note that it is impossible to include every possible cause of pain here, only the more common ones. In the main, we have excluded the discussion of pain caused by injuries other than excessive use.

Before starting your research, it's very important to understand the following key terms, which you will be encountering frequently (see Figure 2). A *joint* is the place where two bones come together for the purpose of motion. The joint is surrounded by a *joint capsule,* which is lined with a layer of cells called the *synovium.* The synovium normally produces a small amount of fluid to lubricate the joint and facilitate movement. When the joint is inflamed, the synovium produces an excessive amount of fluid. The joint becomes warm, tender, swollen, and even red. This is called *synovitis.*

A *muscle* is a body tissue which has the ability to contract or shorten, thereby moving the bones. Excessive use of the muscles can cause *strain* or a small tear in the muscle. Severe muscle inflammation is called *myositis.*

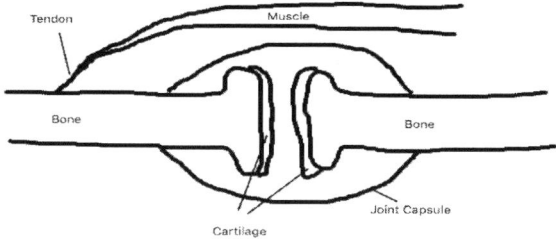

Figure 2 - Cross-Section of a Joint.

Figure 2. Cross-section of a joint. Bone ends are covered with cartilage. Synovium surrounds the joint space and lines the inside of the joint capsule. Muscle terminates in a tendon that attaches to bone.Tendons are fibrous pulleys attaching muscle to bone. These enable the muscles to move the bones. Surrounding the tendon is a sheath, *the lining of which is composed of synovial cells that produce a small amount of fluid. If a tendon becomes inflamed, this is called either* tendonitis *or* tenosynovitis, *the latter term more accurately describing the inflammation effect on the tendon and its sheath.*

A *bone* is a living tissue composed of protein and calcium. This is the framework upon which the body is built. Bony growths can occur near joints, particularly where tendons attach to bone. These bony growths are called *spurs.* Depending upon a spur's size and location, it may cause a great deal of pain in the affected area.

A *bursa* is a small sac that separates muscles and their tendons from other muscles and bone. The inner lining of these sacs also consists of synovial cells. When these become inflamed, the condition is called *bursitis.*

A nerve acts as an electrical wire to bring messages to and from the brain. A nerve can be either *motor, sensory,* or both. A *motor nerve* might, for example, tell a muscle to contract upon a command from the brain. A *sensory nerve* might tell the brain that a part of the body has been injured. If this injury is bad enough, the brain will read this "message" as pain.

A *ligament* is a fibrous tissue that attaches bone to bone. These are supporting tissues that give stability to various body parts. A tear of a ligament is called a *sprain*.

Certain basic disease processes affecting multiple body areas will be mentioned repeatedly in the following pages; they bear description here to remind you of the terminology. These are the *CORE* diseases—diseases affecting the joints. CORE stands for crystal diseases, osteoarthritis, rheumatoid arthritis as well as other connective tissue diseases, and enthesopathies.

The crystal *diseases* include *gout, pseudogout,* and other diseases that provoke joint inflammation through the formation of microscopic crystals in the joint fluid.

Osteoarthritis is degenerative joint disease (also called "wear and tear" arthritis), although it is not really certain whether overuse actually causes it. This is the most common form of arthritis and is often associated with spur formation.

Rheumatoid arthritis and related connective tissue diseases are autoimmune diseases for, in most cases, they produce antibodies that seem to be directed against the body itself. It is uncertain what causes these diseases, though genetic research is providing some important answers. It is known, however, that they can produce a great deal of inflammation in the joints. The other connective tissue diseases include *lupus erythematosus, scleroderma, polymyositis, Sjögren's syndrome,* and overlap syndromes in which two or more of these connective tissue diseases occur together.

Enthesopathy, the last element of CORE, is also called *spondyloarthropathy.* This group of diseases includes *ankylosing spondylitis, psoriatic arthritis,* the various forms of *arthritis associated with inflammatory bowel disease*, and *reactive arthropathy.* The *enthesis* is any attachment to bone, either ligament or tendon. These structures tend to become inflamed with enthesopathies; however, these diseases can involve the joints directly as well.

For a more detailed discussion of the CORE diseases, please turn to chapter 8.

The Foot

All of us have experienced at least some degree of foot discomfort. This appendage bears the brunt of our weight and so is subject to enormous stresses, whether we are walking, running, or even standing still. Figure 3 illustrates some causes of pain in the foot.

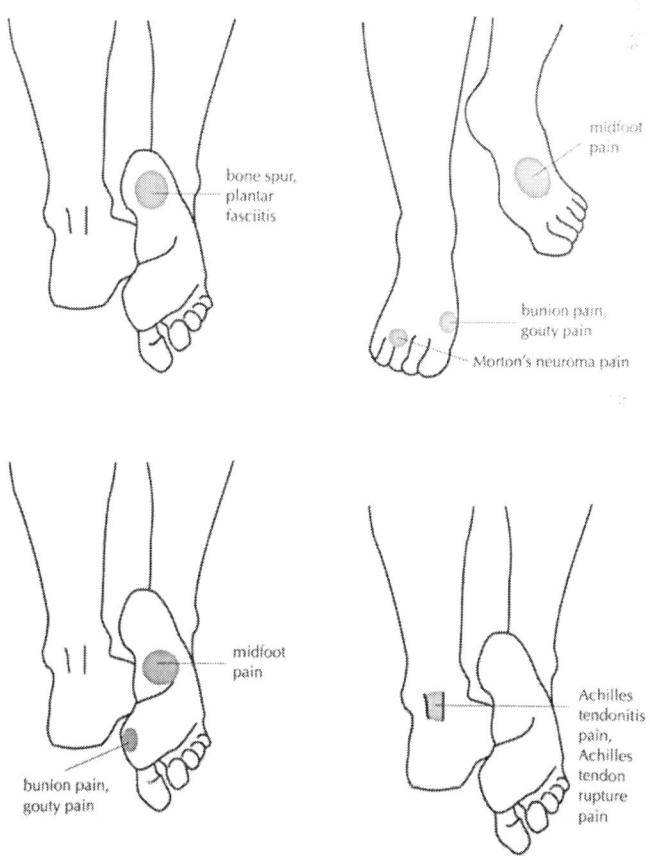

Figure 3. Painful areas on the foot.

If you're experiencing pain on the bottom of your heel as you walk, you might be suffering from a *bony spur,* which may be occurring secondarily to *osteoarthritis, rheumatoid arthritis,* or an *enthesopathy.* Pain of the bottom of the heel, particularly when you are just starting to walk, may be due to fasciitis, an inflammation of the tough fibrous tissue on the bottom of the foot. *Plantar (sole) fasciitis* is associated with flat feet, *spurs, enthesopathy, rheumatoid arthritis, sarcoidosis,* and *fluoride* pill treatment.

Midfoot pain occurs when you walk and involves the middle section of the foot, involving either the top of the foot, the bottom, or both. Pain on the top of the foot can be due to *tendinopathy* or a *bony spur.* A *march fracture* is an actual bone break caused by too much walking. It is a common occurrence among Army recruits. In this case, there is severe tenderness in the middle and front of the foot.

Another cause of midfoot pain (as well as pain to the front of the foot) is joint destruction associated with *diabetes mellitus.* For unclear reasons, when diabetes (or other related diseases) destroys the nerve supply to a joint, the joint is disrupted, resulting in what is called a *Charcot's joint.*

Finally, a potential cause for pain in the midfoot is *osteomyelitis* or infection of the bone. This usually occurs from an object piercing the skin and depositing bacteria into the bony substance itself.

There are many causes for pain in the front of the foot. If you have pain between your third and fourth toes, you may have a Morton's *neuroma,* a trapped nerve that occurs most commonly in middle-aged women. With this complaint, you will feel pain regardless of whether you are standing, sitting, or lying down, and you may experience numbness, burning, and aching, particularly in the fourth toe. If you have this problem you may have found that your only relief comes from massaging the toes and the front of the foot.

Pain in the front of the foot may also be the result of obvious structural changes such as *hammer toes* and *bunions.* A *bunion* is a bursa at the base of the large toe. It is very often associated with an outward deviation of the big toe called *hallux valgus*. This deviation may be genetic in origin, or it can be a manifestation of either *rheumatoid arthritis* or *osteoarthritis*. Patients experiencing these structural changes have a great deal of difficulty wearing high heels or constricting shoes.

There are multiple small joints in the front of the foot which can cause a great deal of discomfort. For example, these joints can be affected by the CORE diseases as well as by an underactive thyroid gland *(hypothyroidism)*. The base of the great toe is particularly prone to gout, which will cause swelling in the joint, redness, and exquisite tenderness in this area. If you experience a great deal of fatigue and aching with standing and walking, you may suffer from pes *planus* or flat feet. Flat feet may also cause ankle pain (see below).

Cold feet, particularly when exposed to cold temperatures, accompanied by a change of color in the foot, may indicate *Raynaud's phenomenon*. This occurs when small arteries (blood vessels) in your feet or hands decrease the blood flow because of *spasm*—that is, the muscular artery tightens up, decreasing the diameter of the vessel and reducing the blood flow. Smoking and certain medications may aggravate the loss of blood flow. *Raynaud's phenomenon* may also be associated with an underlying connective tissue disease.

The cause of foot numbness, tingling, and burning is not usually "poor circulation" as most people tend to believe. If you have these sensations in the entire foot or in the soles (partially or entirely), you may have what is called a *peripheral neuropathy*. Patients complain of "cardboard" or "stiff" feet. These abnormal sensations can also be present in a part of the lower leg. This is caused by the abnormal function of the sensory nerves in the feet. With peripheral neuropathy, there is involvement of all the tiny sensory nerves in the skin over a fairly diffuse area—for example, the entire foot. More localized nerve involvement may occur when a large nerve is trapped by soft tissue or bone, which produces aching, burning, tingling, or numbness in particular areas of the foot.

If these sensations are present in the sole and the inner aspect of the ankle, you may have *tarsal tunnel syndrome* which is compression of the tibial nerve near the inner ankle.

A pinched nerve in the low back may produce pain, numbness, tingling, and burning in the sole and outer aspect of the foot. This may occur when a disc in the low back ruptures, pressing on the nerve roots and causing sciatica

If your foot swells, a number of different conditions may be responsible. *Reflex sympathetic dystrophy syndrome, crystal diseases,* over activity of the thyroid gland *(hyperthyroidism),* low body protein, and poor function of the leg veins may be the cause.

The Ankle

The ankle is composed of two joints surrounded by tendons that enable us to move the foot. One joint allows for the movement of the foot up and down; the other permits the heel to turn inward and outward. Foot movement, then, is very involved, and the ankle, as the conductor of the body weight to the foot, is prone to physical stress- related injury and disease, such as *Achilles tendinopathy* and *sprains.*

Achilles tendinopathy manifests as pain at the back of the heel. Another cause for inflammation there is a *bony spur,* produced by either *osteoarthritis* or *enthesopathies,* which may rub against and irritate the tendon. This tendon may itself become inflamed by *crystal diseases, enthesopathies, rheumatoid arthritis,* any one of the other connective tissue diseases, or may be associated with *hyperlipidemia* (elevated blood cholesterol or triglycerides). Statin medications for cholesterol and quinolone antibiotics may also cause Achilles tendonopathy.

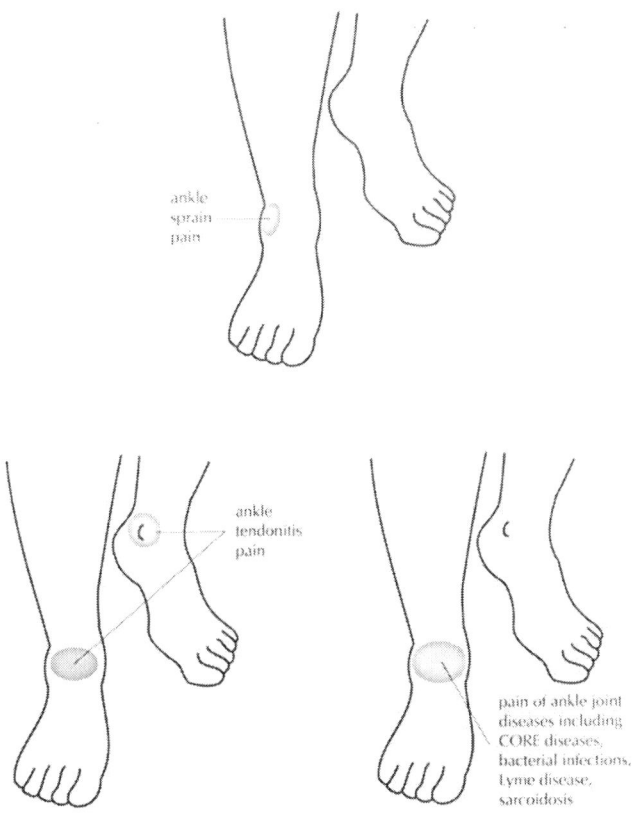

ankle
sprain
pain

ankle
tendonitis
pain

pain of ankle joint
diseases including
CORE diseases,
bacterial infections,
Lyme disease,
sarcoidosis

Figure 4. Areas of pain likely to occur in the ankle.

At times, the cause of Achilles tendon disorders is unclear. People with active Achilles tendinopathy tend to walk on their toes to decrease the tension on the tendon. A tendon can become tight—and subsequently uncomfortable—from wearing high heels or from not walking for a long period of time, as is the case with bedridden patients. Tendinopathy may simply be caused by the shoes, which may be rubbing against the Achilles tendon (such is the cost of the choice between comfort and style). In most of these cases, lifting the toes will cause pain at the back of the heel.

Lastly, the Achilles tendon can rupture. Here, you may actually hear and feel the snap before experiencing pain and difficulty in walking or standing on the toes. The cause of *Achilles tendon rupture* may be a sudden trauma, often sports related. An Achilles tendon is more prone to rupture if it has been inflamed, chronically irritated or had cortisone injected into it.

Along with the Achilles, a fair number of tendons pass over the ankle to manipulate the foot. Any one or a number of these tendons may cause pain and swelling. Ankle *tendinopathy* may be the result of excessive use or bad shoes. It may also be caused by *rheumatoid arthritis* and other connective tissue diseases, *crystal disease,* and *enthesopathies.* Finally, ankle tendinopathy may be the result of still other diseases, including *sarcoidosis* and *gonorrhea. Sarcoidosis* is an inflammatory systemic disease of unclear cause that can affect the lungs, skin, eyes, bones, and joints. It is treatable.

Another frequent cause of ankle pain is an ankle ligament tear commonly called a sprain, which generally occurs on the outside of the ankle. You may remember twisting the ankle badly in one direction or another. A significant *sprain* may make the ankle feel unnaturally loose, giving it a tendency to "give way." A sprain may also result in swelling or an *ecchymosis* ("black and blue mark"). People who have flat feet often suffer from ligament stretching and tearing because the flat foot causes an outward deviation of the heel. This leads to excess stress on the ligaments as well as on the ankle joints themselves.

If you have not injured your ankle but are still experiencing severe swelling, redness, and pain, one or both of the ankles may be afflicted with any one of the CORE diseases. Certain infections, particularly *Lyme disease* and various *bacterial infections* (including *gonorrhea),* can all affect the ankle. Immediate diagnosis of ankle infection is important, because an infected ankle may result in severe and permanent damage. *Sarcoidosis* may also involve the ankle.

When ankle swelling is not associated with pain but is simply a "tight" feeling, it may be due to fluid excess or *edema* in the lower leg and foot. The most common cause of edema is poor functioning of the veins in the legs. When this occurs, there is a backlog of fluid in the lower legs, particularly after prolonged standing or having the feet hang down without support.

One basic thing to watch for is this: Edema tends to involve the lower leg and the entire foot while arthritis and tendinopathy are usually confined to the ankle itself.

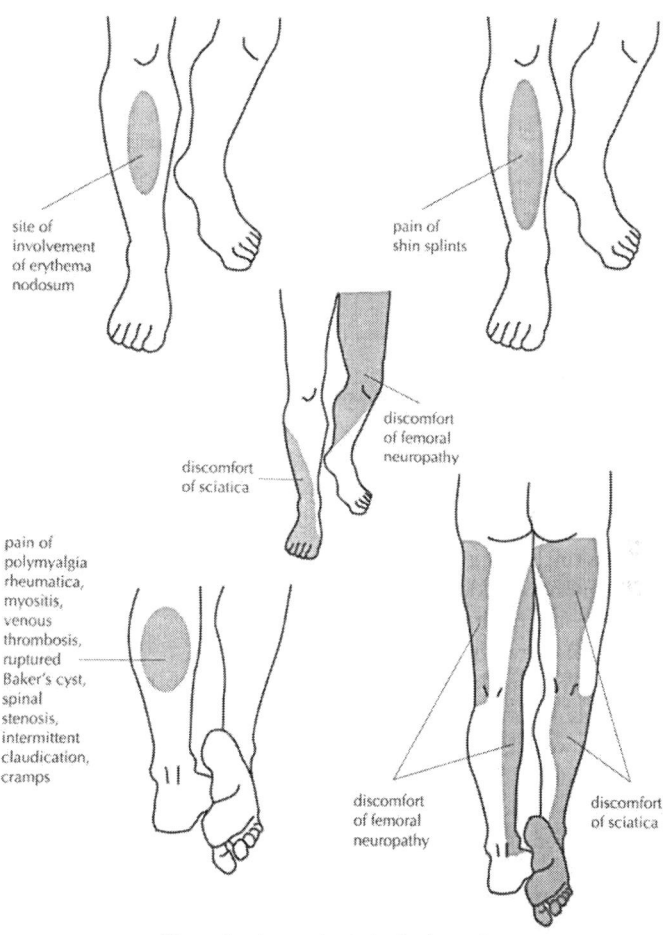

site of
involvement
of erythema
nodosum

pain of
shin splints

discomfort
of femoral
neuropathy

discomfort
of sciatica

pain of
polymyalgia
rheumatica,
myositis,
venous
thrombosis,
ruptured
Baker's cyst,
spinal
stenosis,
intermittent
claudication,
cramps

discomfort
of femoral
neuropathy

discomfort
of sciatica

Figure 5. Areas of pain in the lower leg.

The Lower Leg

For our purposes, the lower leg is the area between the knee and the ankle. Generally, pain in this part of the body is restricted to one of three areas: the shin, the calf, or the entire lower leg. Figure 5 illustrates some common painful areas of the lower leg.

If the front of your lower leg hurts, particularly after running or walking, you may be suffering from *shin splints*. This is a fairly common but poorly understood problem that results from excessive activity following a period of inactivity. Most experts believe that the condition is the result of tiny tears occurring where the muscle in the shin area attaches to the bone. Usually located in the front and inner aspects of the lower leg, the pain can last from hours to days. A short rest period may not be sufficient to alleviate the pain, although the overall treatment includes long periods of rest.

Paget's disease, a condition in which there is an abnormal remodeling of the bony structure, may also affect the lower leg, causing pain.

Pain in the back of the lower leg or the calf may be the result of a number of causes. *Polymyalgia rheumatica* may first appear as an achy stiffness in the calf muscle, particularly in the morning. There is no pain to the touch. Subsequent symptoms may include soreness on both sides of the body, often involving the thighs, the groins, as well as the upper arms and shoulders. Polymyalgia rheumatica is a treatable, if little understood, low-grade inflammation of the muscles.

Another cause of inflammation of the muscles is *myositis* or *polymyositis*. This is a severe muscle inflammation that occurs in the thigh and other densely muscled areas of the body. In this condition, the upper arms, thighs, and perhaps the calves become extremely weak. Walking, climbing stairs, even standing up become difficult. The muscles may be tender to the touch.

Another cause of severe pain—one with potentially fatal

consequences—is the formation of blood clots in the calf, particularly in the deeper veins *(venous thrombosis)*. This can result in the swelling of the calf and lower leg. Pain is significant, particularly when you lift your toes. The danger with such blood clots is that they can embolize—that is, move to various parts of the body, including the lung, with sometimes catastrophic results.

A ruptured *Baker's cyst,* which bears some clinical resemblance to a blood clot may also cause pain in the calf. A *Baker's cyst* is a bursa behind the knee which becomes enlarged and inflamed. This condition often occurs with any type of knee arthritis of long duration. The bursa can eventually rupture, causing pain and swelling. When this happens, walking becomes extremely painful.

There are several other possible causes of pain in the calf when walking. One is *spinal stenosis,* which occurs when the spinal cord in the low back is pinched as a result of a narrowing of the spinal canal—through the development within the canal of *bony spurs, scar tissue, ruptured discs,* or any combination of these pressing against the cord. With this condition, you may experience back pain which travels down the entire leg, usually on both sides. You may feel numbness and weakness, particularly with walking. Walking becomes limited as the discomfort increases. People with spinal stenosis tend to stop walking, sit down, and lean forward. This posture eases the pressure on the spinal cord and alleviates the discomfort. A pinched nerve or nerve damage in the back may cause discomfort in the lower leg. *Sciatica,* a pinching of the lower nerve roots in the low back, may cause numbness, tingling, burning, and pain in the lower leg, particularly the calf and outer aspect of the lower leg. *Femoral neuropathy* may cause similar sensations in the front and inner aspects of the lower leg. Femoral neuropathy may be caused by *diabetes* or it may be caused by a pinching of the nerve roots of the femoral nerve—for example, by a ruptured disc.

Another cause of pain, particularly with walking, is poor circulation. Artery disease of the lower legs can cause pain in the calves, even after walking only a short distance. One or both calves may be affected. This is called *intermittent claudication,* and it only occurs when the muscles of the calves are exercised. As the requirement for blood flow increases, the arteries are not capable of delivering because of artery disease and narrowing. Patients with this problem often stop walking to "window shop." In fact, they are really resting their muscles to lessen the pain. This is somewhat similar to a case where angina develops with exercise because narrowed blood vessels pass an inadequate blood flow to the heart muscle.

An aspect of the blood flow problem is the cramping, which is indistinguishable from other types of cramp except insofar as the affected area responds well to rest. If you are suffering from *cramps,* particularly at night, you are not alone. Cramps of the calf is a very common form of discomfort known as a "charley horse." These knots occur in the back of the calf, especially when resting in bed. Generally, excessive activity or electrolyte abnormalities cause this kind of pain. Poor circulation, as mentioned, is another potential cause. Whatever the case, cramps are usually quite treatable.

If you suffer from pain or discomfort in the entire lower leg, you may be experiencing *peripheral neuropathy.* This is a situation in which the nerves do not function properly over such extended areas as the foot and the lower leg. This disease is often manifested through tingling, numbness, and burning. Peripheral neuropathy often comes as a result of *diabetes.* At times, the affected area can be exquisitely sensitive even to the lightest touch.

Then there is *restless leg syndrome,* also referred to as *periodic extremity movement disorder,* where patients experience continuous movement of their legs, especially when they are trying to sleep. Though not usually particularly painful, restless leg syndrome is uncomfortable, and leaves the legs feeling heavy and tired. It is unclear precisely what causes this problem, but many experts feel that a central mechanism, perhaps in the brain tissue itself, is responsible for the electrical impulses that prompt the legs to move about. This is, fortunately, a treatable condition.

Hypertrophic osteoarthropathy is a condition that may be responsible for a deep, aching sensation in the long bones, particularly in the lower legs when standing or whenever the legs are in a dependent position below the level of the heart. With this condition, the bones thicken. Likewise, the fingertips may also thicken, a sign called "clubbing" that gives the finger a drumstick appearance. Hypertrophic osteoarthropathy and clubbing may be idiopathic; that is, they may be of unclear origin. They can appear in association with a wide spectrum of illnesses that seem to have nothing to do with the legs, among them emphysema, lung tumors, cystic fibrosis, alcoholic liver disease, and heart valve infections. Because of the extreme discomfort when the legs are in a dependent position, patients with hypertrophic osteoarthropathy tend to elevate the legs to reduce their discomfort.

Occasionally, pain in the lower leg can be directly linked to small nodules or lumps on the calf or shin. These can be red, warm, and very tender. This is a manifestation of the inflammation of the blood vessel, which may, in turn, be related to fatty tissue inflammation. One of the more common types of nodules formed in such cases is called *erythema nodosum*. This refers to the red lumps, and these may signify any one of a large variety of illnesses. Erythema nodosum usually improves by itself, but the condition can become chronic. If you develop such nodules on the lower leg, you really should visit your physician.

The Knee

One of the difficulties engineers faced in designing the artificial knee was duplicating the extraordinary complexity of the knee joint. This consists of three different compartments. From the front, the knee has a medial (inner) and lateral (outer) compartment, each separated by a *meniscus* (a kind of shock absorber). From the side, one can see that there is a third compartment right behind the knee cap. The structure of the knee also involves several bursal sacs. It's no wonder, then, that given its complexity and what we expect it to do, the knee is subject to a wide variety of problems, many of which can be extremely painful. Figure 6 illustrates painful areas in the knee. If you find that your knee is locking when you try to move it or if it is buckling as you walk, you may have an internal derangement— damage to the intricate mechanism of the knee. Perhaps you feel a snapping sensation or hear a popping as you bend it. The culprit may be a tear in the meniscus or perhaps a loose body—called a "joint mouse," usually a bony particle— in one of the compartments. Or, it may be a plica, where the inner lining of the knee *(synovium)* has a fold which has become inflamed. All of these problems can be extremely painful and cause the knee to swell.

Other causes of pain in the knee include *osteoarthritis.* Knee pain may also occur when the ligaments surrounding the knee develop a tear *(sprain).*

Anserine bursitis frequently strikes women. This bursitis occurs on the inner aspect of the knee toward the front, approximately an inch below the kneecap. This often occurs in overweight middle-aged women and causes pain when climbing stairs and is even present at rest. Often, walking alleviates the discomfort. Women may be prone to develop this in the right knee, as they tend to keep their knees together and exert an outward force when using the gas pedal of a car. Exerting force with the leg in an outward direction while keeping the knees together puts stress on the anserine bursa. Fortunately, this condition can be easily treated.

People commonly complain of pain in the front of the knee. They often speak of "grinding" behind the kneecap and experience sharp pain with standing up or going up stairs. The problem is cartilage damage behind the kneecap and can affect both young and middle-aged people. Known in the past as *chondromalacia patellae,* the modern term for this problem is *patellofemoral dysfunction* and describes any problem involving the compartment behind the kneecap.

Pain located directly at the bottom of the kneecap and extending down a short distance to the top of the shin may be due to *patellar tendonitis also known as* "Jumper's knee".

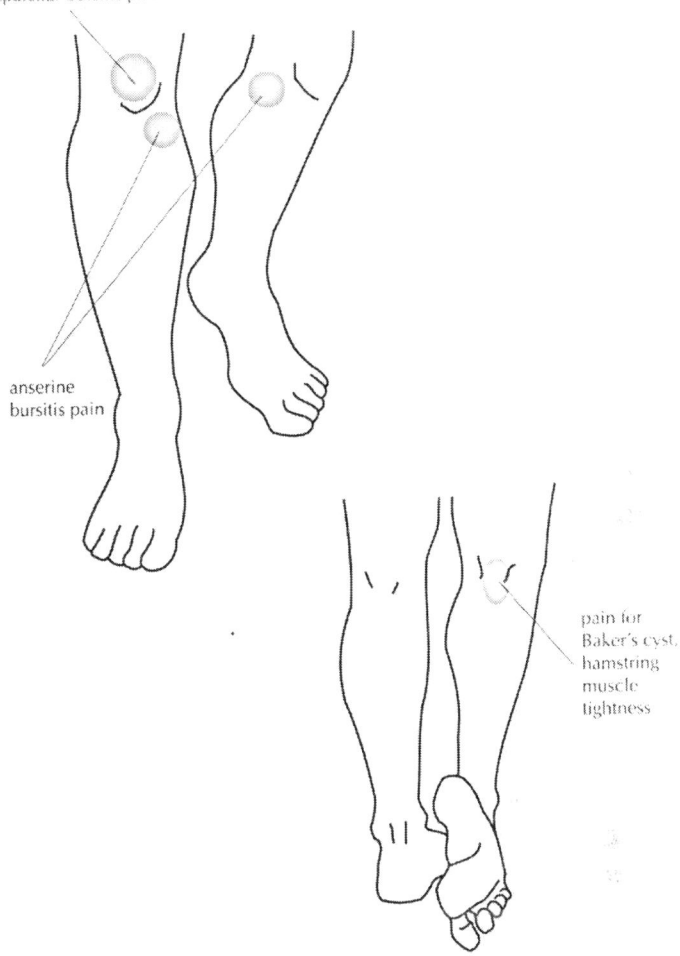

Figure 6. Areas of pain in the knee.

Occasionally, a patient will complain of pain directly in front of the kneecap. The *prepatellar bursa* is located there and may become inflamed. This is the called "housemaid's knee," and can affect any adult who spends a lot of time on his or her hands and knees.

A potential cause for pain behind the knee is a *Baker's cyst,* also called a *popliteal cyst.* It is a bursa (pocket) behind the knee with an opening that allows fluid from the knee to flow into the bursa.

Eventually, the bursa distends. It can rupture into the calf, imitating the kind of pain and swelling associated with *phlebitis* (vein inflammation) or even a blood clot *(venous thrombosis).* Any chronic knee arthritis may lead to this condition. The patient often feels a sensation of "fullness" behind the knee and a chronic aching in this area.

Other causes of pain behind the knee include *hamstring muscle tightness* and inflammation or degeneration of another structure called the popliteal tendon

The knee is a particular target for the CORE diseases *(Crystal diseases, Osteoarthritis, Rheumatoid arthritis* and *other connective tissue diseases,* as well as *Enthesopathy;* see chapter 8). Any one of these attacking the knee may cause swelling. Infections such as *Lyme disease, gonorrhea, tuberculosis,* or other *bacteria* may also attack the knee.

Other conditions such as hyperlipidemia (elevated blood cholesterol or triglycerides) *sarcoidosis* and *hemochromatosis* (iron overload disease) can cause knee problems.

Diabetes mellitus may lead to severe joint destruction due to disruption of the nerve supply to the knee. This results in a *Charcot's joint.* Either an underactive *(hypothyroid)* or overactive *(hyperthyroid)* thyroid gland may cause knee stiffness and swelling.

Despite the complexity of the joint, conservative treatment can alleviate most knee problems. As in all cases, however, the precise diagnosis is essential for determining the most effective treatment.

The Thigh

The thigh, located between the torso and the lower leg, may develop pain due to either hip or back disease. At the top of the thigh is the hip joint. Hip disorders may present as pain or weakness in the thigh or groin.

Nerves originating in the spinal cord pass through the thigh to the lower leg and foot. Pressure on a nerve or nerve root in the back may cause pain in the thigh or lower leg. Figure 7 illustrates areas of pain in the thigh.

Given the complicated interrelation of the thigh to the lower back and hips, knowing where you experience pain in the thigh will often help determine the original source of the problem.

The Back of the Thigh

Hamstring muscles are located in the back of the thigh and tightness is usually the result of a lack of exercise and loss of flexibility of these muscles. A *hamstring pull* or *strain* occurs with stretching and sometimes tearing of the hamstring muscle. Both hamstring tightness and pulls may produce pain. A *blood clot* or *venous thrombosis* can sometimes present as pain in the back of the thigh.

A disc disorder or a spur (a bony arthritic growth) in the low back may compress a nerve root, causing pain to travel down the back of the thigh, often with simultaneous low back pain. This condition is frequently described as *sciatica.*

The Front of the Thigh

Pain in the front of the thigh also may be the result of nerve compression in the back, but at a slightly higher level than the sciatic nerve. The sciatic nerve originates in the lower spine. The *femoral nerve* has its roots a few inches above the sciatic nerve in the low back and travels down the front of the thigh. The femoral nerve can be affected by *diabetes,* causing pain or weakness in the front of the thigh.

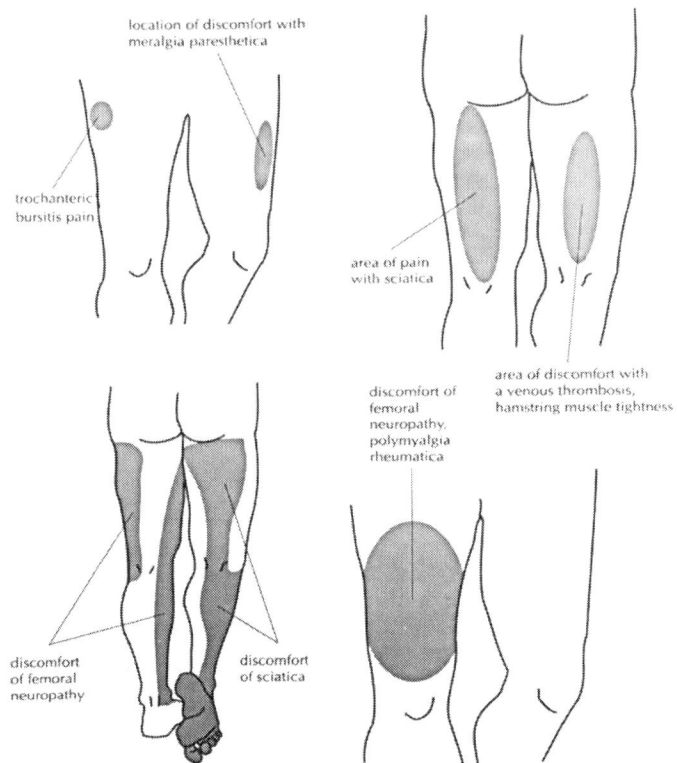

Figure 7. Areas of pain in the thigh.

As a result, the thigh is often the site of *pain referral* or *radiation*. In other words, we often feel pain in a place where it does not originate.

Another potential cause of pain in the front of the thigh is *polymyalgia rheumatica,* an inflammatory condition that causes muscle aching and stiffness in multiple areas including the thigh.

Finally, the anterior thigh is composed of a large mass of muscle, and muscle diseases may first present as problems in the thigh. This may present as pain and/or weakness particularly when getting up from a chair or going up stairs.

The Outside of the Thigh

Pain on the outside of the thigh may be the result of a number of origins. Sciatica, while it most directly involves the back of the thigh, may cause pain down the outside of the thigh as well. The *trochanteric bursa,* located in the upper outside thigh area, may become inflamed, causing pain to shoot down the outside of the thigh. When inflamed, this bursa is tender, particularly at night. Patients suffering with this condition often have difficulty sleeping on the side of bursitis. There are also several tendons, such as the gluteus medius, in this area that may become damaged (tendinopathy) and be the source of the pain.

Numbness, tingling, pain, as well as a sense of burning in the outer aspect of the thigh (and perhaps the front as well), may be due to a condition called *meralgia paresthetica*. In this condition, one of the superficial nerves of the thigh becomes compressed at the point where it emerges into the thigh. This occurs particularly as a result of weight gain, such as with pregnancy, but it may also occur in *diabetes*. A person may experience more pain when walking or standing than when sitting, and the pain may be intermittent, as the nerve may be compressed only from time to time.

Pain in the Entire Thigh

Pain in the entire thigh may result from *polymyalgia rheumatica* (described above) or *polymyositis*. Polymyositis is a severe inflammatory disease that affects many muscles in the body, causing inflammation so severe that it can permanently damage muscle tissue. This disease often affects the thighs because some of the largest muscles in the body are located here. However, the predominant clinical problem with polymyositis is weakness rather than pain.

Another cause for pain in the entire thigh might be neurologic damage associated with diabetes or *diabetic neuropathy*. This may cause burning, weakness, numbness, tingling, and increased pain.

Spinal stenosis is another possible cause of pain in the entire thigh. This can cause pain and/or weakness, particularly when walking. In this condition the spinal cord is compressed by arthritis and degenerated discs inside the spinal canal. Such pain most often occurs with walking and decreases with stopping, sitting, stooping, or leaning forward.

Several sources of bone diseases should be considered when evaluating thigh pain, especially when the pain is restricted to one rather than both thighs. An example might be a malignancy. However, a bony tumor pressing on the spinal cord may cause pain in both thighs. Because the femur is a very large bone, it is potentially subject to a number of bone diseases. *Paget's disease* typically manifests as a sharp or dull pain in the thigh, aggravated by walking. Paget's can affect any bone in the body, and is the result of defective bone modeling which, in turn, produces imperfect bone. While this irregular bone may be a source of significant pain, it only rarely degenerates into a malignancy. Occasionally, the bone produced with Paget's is so abnormal that it may fracture or break upon standing up.

A *metastatic tumor* is one that originates in one location and then spreads. *Prostate and breast* cancer, along with certain other tumors, have a tendency to spread in this fashion. Should any of these tumors spread to the thigh bone, the resultant pain may be the first indication that something is awry.

Another condition your doctor might take into account is osteomyelitis, an infection of the bony substance itself. This occurs if infectious bacteria reach the bone, either through a deep wound or via the bloodstream.

Finally, a fracture of the femur (thigh bone) is very painful, and people are often unaware of exactly what has happened. Occasionally, a patient may experience a fracture without falling, especially if the bone is thin—a result of *osteoporosis*—or weakened by other bony conditions, such as vitamin D deficiency, Paget's disease, bony tumors, long term use of bisphosphonate drugs used to treat osteoporosis, or congenital disease affecting bone formation.

The Buttocks and Groin

If you are feeling pain in the buttocks, you may be suffering from *ischial bursitis,* otherwise known as *tailor's bottom.* With this condition, your pelvic bone comes into contact with the surface which you are sitting on. A small bursal sac on each side of the buttocks becomes inflamed, particularly after prolonged sitting on a firm surface.

Another potential cause for pain in the buttocks is *pain referral* or *radiation*—that is, a neurologic problem in one area that manifests itself elsewhere (such as *sciatica*). Figure 8 illustrates painful areas in the buttocks and groin.

Pain in the groin has several possible causes—hip diseases, for example. Osteoarthritis of the hip often presents with groin discomfort. Patients may complain about the inability to get their shoes and socks on and off because of limited motion and because of pain. Pain may radiate from an arthritic or fixed *sacroiliac joint* into the groin. The sacroiliac joints are located on both sides of the low back approximately an inch and a half above the tailbone. Another and perhaps more obvious cause for pain in this region of the body is a groin muscle pull. Such pulls or strains can occur in the middle-aged "weekend warrior" as well as in the seasoned athlete. *Hernias* often

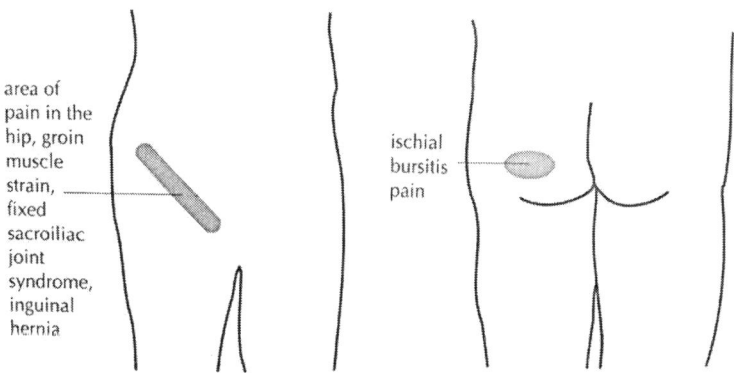

Figure 8. Painful areas in the buttocks and groin.

produce discomfort in the groin area. In such cases, you may feel a groin bulge when you are bearing down (as when you are attempting to move your bowels). Finally, pain in the groin may also result from *polymyalgia rheumatica* (described above).

The Hips

The hip joint is a ball and socket joint formed by the thigh bone (the femur) and the pelvic bone. The round head of the femur allows for a wide range of movement. A number of conditions affecting the hip joint cause pain when walking or standing up and often manifest as pain in the groin. Figure 9 illustrates painful areas of the hips.

Along with the CORE diseases, hip pain may be due to a destructive process called *avascular necrosis.* In this condition, part of the bone actually dies. Using cortisone derivatives (corticosteroids or "steroids") over an extended period of time or having *sickle cell anemia* can predispose a person to develop aseptic necrosis. Current research indicates that this condition is due to a decrease in blood flow in the hip joint.

An overactive thyroid gland *(hyperthyroid)* may cause hip pain.

Hemochromatosis, or iron overload disease, is another condition which can involve the hip joint.

Hip pain may also be the result of infection in the hip joint itself. Various *bacteria* can invade and possibly destroy the hip joint. In such cases, a person may experience fever and find that any movement of the hip is very painful. The microorganism may be introduced inadvertently during a hip injection or it may reach the hip via the bloodstream.

An obvious cause of hip pain is a stress fracture following a fall, particularly in the elderly who already suffer from *osteoporosis* or thinning of the bone. *Bony tumors* may similarly cause pain in the hip and can arise from the bone or, more commonly, metastasize or migrate from a remote tumor.

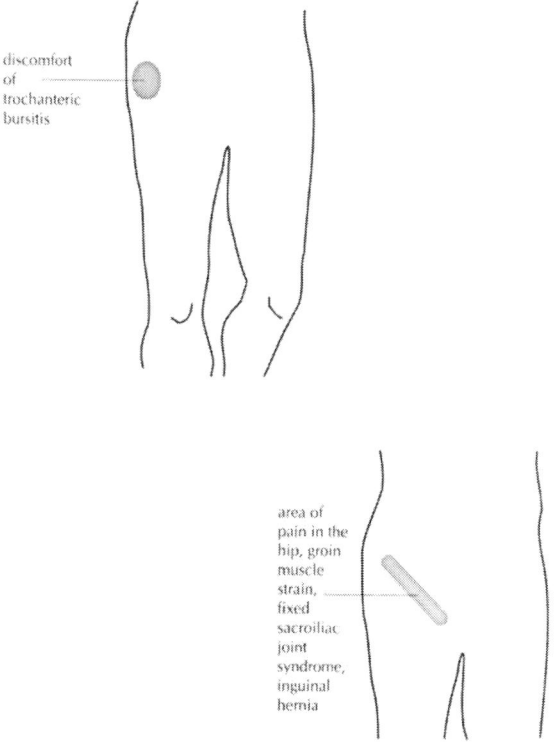

discomfort
of
trochanteric
bursitis

area of
pain in the
hip, groin
muscle
strain,
fixed
sacroiliac
joint
syndrome,
inguinal
hernia

Figure 9. Painful areas in the hips.

Paget's disease, a condition in which there is an abnormal remodeling of bone, may cause hip pain by involving the femur or pelvic bones. It may do so by producing enough faulty bone so that a fracture (break) occurs, or simply by transforming enough normal bone into defective bone. Rarely, bone involved with Paget's disease may evolve into a bony tumor.

Problems in the back can radiate to the groin. Discs pressing against a nerve root and similar structural problems in the spine may manifest as pain in the groin. If arthritic change strikes the sacroiliac joint, the resultant *fixed sacroiliac joint syndrome* can introduce pain directly into the groin. *Fixed sacroiliac joint syndrome* occurs when arthritis (often *osteoarthritis)* decreases movement in the sacroiliac joint, causing low back pain and pain in the groin as well as the inner thigh. Treatment, usually in the form of physical therapy, is aimed at mobilizing the affected joint.

Kidney stones can often cause pain in the groin. An inguinal hernia may also cause significant groin discomfort. Muscle disease can affect the hip as well. *Polymyalgia rheumatica,* may cause stiffness and aching in the groin.

The groin is also susceptible to muscle strain (note: ligaments are sprained; muscles are strained). Muscle pulls or strains can occur in three degrees: *first degree* is a stretched muscle; *second degree* is a partial tear; third *degree* is a complete tear. Simple muscle pulls often affect the groin.

Pain in the outer aspect of the hip may be caused by a *trochanteric bursitis or trochanteric tendinopathy.* Often for unclear reasons, this bursa becomes inflamed or one of the three tendons in this area may develop tears from degenerative change, particularly in the middle aged and the elderly. The resultant pain occurs in the upper, outer thigh, with walking, climbing, or lying down on the involved hip. The pain can be sudden or can start slowly. In extreme cases, the pain may radiate down the outer aspect of the thigh.

The Low Back

Low back pain is the price human beings pay for the ability to stand and sit upright. Because human beings often find uncomfortable and unsupportive conditions in which to work, injury to the low back is a major cause of disability in the working population. Figure 10 illustrates the areas of pain in the lower back.

The low back consists of bony building blocks, *vertebrae,* which are separated from each other by shock-absorbing discs. The vertebral bodies are attached to one another from behind on each side by paired joints called *facet joints.* Behind the vertebral bodies lies the canal through which the spinal cord travels. Nerve roots branch off the spinal cord at each level of vertebrae and disc.

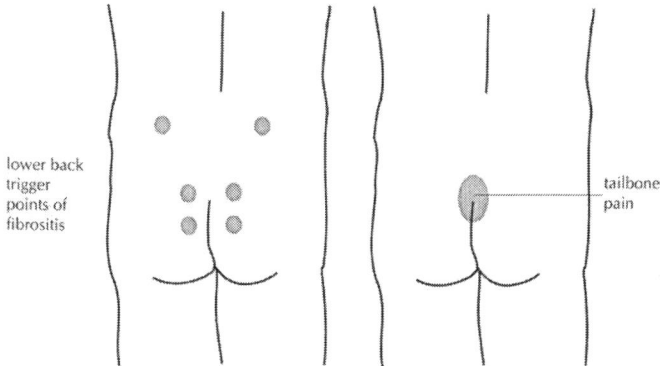

Figure 10. Painful areas in the lower back.

In this enormously complicated mass of flexible bone, nerve, and muscle, it is easy for something to go wrong. A disc or bone may press on the nerves as they leave the spinal canal, causing *sciatica* (shooting pain that travels down the back of the thigh) or *femoral neuropathy,* which causes pain to shoot down the front of the thigh. The resultant pain may be experienced as numbness, tingling, burning, and/or weakness in the thigh and possibly the lower leg.

Simple muscle strain from overuse is a common cause of localized low back pain.

Another problem in the back, which can cause pain to shoot down the leg, particularly when walking, is *spinal stenosis.* Affecting people primarily between the ages of 40 and 70, spinal stenosis occurs when the spinal canal is narrowed by bony spurs, disc herniation, scarring, or enlargement of the ligaments. Any one of these can press directly on the spinal cord, particularly when walking. Further symptoms are lower leg weakness when walking or even standing. Spinal stenosis may cause pain in the low back, the buttocks, as well as in both legs. Resting, sitting, or leaning forward tends to alleviate the pressure on the spinal cord, thereby bringing temporary relief. Patients may respond to epidural steroid injections or physical therapy. Permanent relief is generally attainable through surgery. However, long term results for pain relief with surgery are highly variable.

Another cause of pain in the low back, the *enthesopathies,* may affect the sciatic nerve. These diseases, exemplified by *ankylosing spondylitis,* involve not only the ligaments of the spine but of the sacroiliac joints as well. If the sciatic nerve touches any of the areas inflamed by the enthesopathy, it may result in sciatica. With these diseases, there is often low back stiffness in the morning upon waking up that lessens somewhat with exercise but worsens again later in the day.

Another potential cause of low back pain accompanied by low leg pain and weakness is a tumor involving the lower spinal nerve roots. This is a serious condition which can result in permanent paralysis if not addressed quickly.

While all of these ailments and diseases reflect the complexity of the low back, localized back pain that does not affect the limbs is the most common problem. Such localized back pain has numerous causes. For example, abnormalities in posture can lead to muscle fatigue, particularly in cases of obesity or inactivity, which leads to poor muscle tone. After too much back movement, a ligament may become sprained and cause pain in the low back.

Osteoarthritis also causes localized low back pain, particularly in the facet joints connecting the vertebrae. At times, these facets joints may become locked, leading to a marked decrease in the movement of the spine.

The discs of the back may be a source of pain when they degenerate. A *ruptured* or *herniated disc* may occur after lifting or from other back injury. Part of the soft disc tissue may push out from the center of the disc and compress the nerve root.

Even if the protruding disc material does not press on a nerve root, the degenerating disc itself may cause pain because it has its own nerve supply in its outer areas. The damaged disc loses resilience and is less capable of absorbing shocks, so there is excessive stress on the facet joints in the back. This, in turn, accelerates facet joint osteoarthritis and leads to increased low back pain.

Abnormal bony growth may result in pain, either through pressing on nerves or by themselves. For example, *Paget's disease* produces abnormal bone in the low back region and, as a result, may cause pain. Similarly, tumors originating in or travelling to the low back may be painful. This is particularly true of *prostate cancer,* which can spread to the low back bones if not caught early. The low back may also be a site for *multiple myeloma,* which is a bony tumor originating in the bone marrow substance itself.

Bacterial infections may attack the low back, affecting either bones or discs. Infection may also occur next to the spinal cord *(spinal epidural abscess)* and may compress the spinal cord, producing leg paralysis. *Tuberculosis* is another cause of infection in the back. *Pott's disease,* tuberculous involvement of the spine, was more common in the pre-antibiotic era, but it still is found on occasion.

A fairly common source of sudden low back pain, particularly in elderly women, is a vertebral compression fracture (break) caused by *osteoporosis* or thin bone. Part or all of the vertebral body collapses because of structural weakening through the leaching out of calcium and loss of bony protein. There is permanent loss of height. The severe pain usually lasts four to six weeks, but some people experience continued muscle spasm and lack of movement for years. The patient develops a hunched posture. This worsens with each successive vertebral compression fracture. When severe osteoporosis occurs, it is only moderately responsive to treatment. It is more easily prevented than treated.

Enthesopathies, described above, are also a frequent cause of localized back pain, particularly in such diseases as *ankylosing spondylitis.* Typically affecting men, this chronic disease usually manifests first as

77

stiffness in the low back when the patient is in his early twenties, and later develops into a loss of back movement. The stiffness tends to improve with exercise but recurs later in the day particularly after a prolonged rest period. Fortunately, this disease is responsive to certain medications as well as exercise.

Another of the many causes of low back pain is *polymyalgia rheumatica,* an inflammatory condition of the muscles generally affecting the muscle masses in the thighs, groin, low back, upper arms, shoulders, and neck. A patient with the condition may experience low back stiffness in the morning, though this tends to improve with activity.

Also, low back pain can be caused by a sacroiliac joint where *osteoarthritic spurs* have formed, which can cause the joint to lock, and lead to what is called *fixed sacroiliac joint syndrome.* The resulting pain travels to the groin. Low back pain occurs particularly when you try to cross your legs by placing the ankle on the thigh—the way most men are accustomed to crossing their legs when sitting.

Fibromyalgia also may cause low back pain. This soft tissue disease affects the muscles and the supporting tissues. With this disease, very sensitive nodules, trigger points, form in the low back. When pressed, these nodules may cause pain that travels to various low back locations and even down the leg. While fibromyalgia is still poorly understood, it is both common as well as treatable.

The low back is also subject to pain originating from deeper organs such as the uterus in women, the prostate in men, and kidney stones. Another example, an *aortic aneurysm* (an enlargement of the large artery in the abdomen) may produce pain in the low back.

Another cause of low back discomfort is *tailbone pain.* This is a fairly common problem that usually occurs after injury to the coccyx or tailbone. Occasionally the tailbone at the low end of the spine may be bruised or fractured, and you might have trouble sitting down. Nonsurgical treatment is usually effective in alleviating this discomfort.

Finally, there is *shingles* pain. It causes pain on only one side of the back. The pain may be sharp or burning and is eventually accompanied by a rash consisting of small blisters on a red base. The "chicken pox virus" causes shingles.

The Upper Back

The structure of the upper back is similar to that of the lower back, but since the upper back supports less weight, it is a less frequent site of back pain. As a general rule of thumb, however, a number of the problems described in the section on the lower back also apply here. Figure 11 illustrates areas of pain in the upper back.

If you experience stiffness and aching, for example, and feel tenderness near the shoulder blades, you may be suffering from *fibromyalgia*, in which trigger points develop in the soft tissues. When pressed, these points cause a stinging, radiant pain. This disease can be localized (upper back) or generalized (the entire back, chest, neck, etc.), and can spread if left untreated. Fortunately, it usually responds to treatment.

The upper back may also be a site of a vertebral body compression fracture due to *osteoporosis*, a disease in which the bone thins. This disease is diffuse, but is most often evident in the large bones and "weak" areas that withstand the stress of weight and motion (the hip, for example, or the vertebrae in the spine). The disease most often affects elderly Caucasian women who have already lost much of their bony mass. The first indication of the condition is usually a sudden pain which travels around the chest on one or both sides to the front. Unfortunately, osteoporosis may worsen with or without treatment.

Another cause of sharp upper back pain which often occurs on one side is *shingles*. The distinctive rash of this ailment may not be apparent initially. However, it may be foreshadowed by a severe sharp and burning pain, followed within a day or two by the appearance of a clear, tiny bleb, or blister, with a red base on the skin. Shingles is caused by the same virus which causes chicken pox.

While cases of *osteoarthritis* are frequent, the disease itself rarely causes upper back pain, perhaps because the upper back does not carry the full weight of the torso and is not subject to the same measures of stress experienced in the low back.

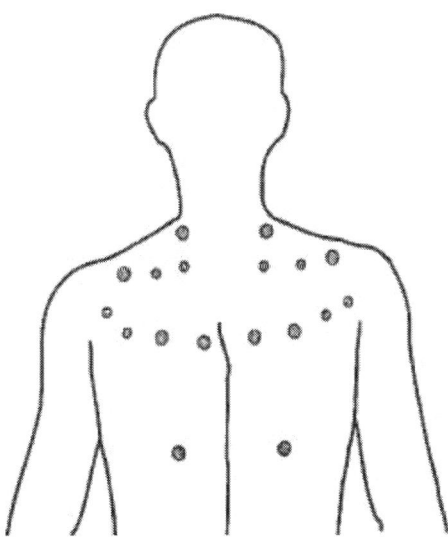

Figure 13 - Areas of Pain in the Upper Back

Upper back trigger points of fibromyalgia

Because of the position of organs in the body cavity, internal diseases may make themselves felt in the upper back. A tumor from a lung or breast cancer which has metastasized or traveled to the bone (ribs and shoulder blade) may initially cause severe pain in the upper back. Similarly, *pleurisy* may show itself as a sharp pain in the upper back when you draw in a deep breath. Pleurisy occurs when the outer lining of the lungs becomes inflamed as the result of various diseases, including pneumonia, virus infection, tuberculosis, and various connective tissue diseases, particularly lupus.

A final cause of upper back pain may be referred pain—that is, pain which travels to an area other than its source. Gallbladder disease, for example, may manifest as pain at the tip of the shoulder blade, especially when taking a deep breath.

The Head

The head isn't just the housing for the brain. It is, in fact, a complex arrangement of different tissues and structures. Muscle covers the entire face and head, allowing us to chew food, move our eyes, furrow our foreheads, and smile in contentment. All these muscles are subject to fatigue, stretching, and pain from overuse. The primary joints in the head are the paired temporomandibular joints that join the lower jaw to the skull. These very active joints are not immune to the same diseases that befall other joints in the body. Inflammation within airspaces in the facial bones, the sinus cavities, may be a source of vexation for millions of allergy sufferers. The numerous blood vessels in the head may become inflamed, constricted, or enlarged, causing circulation problems which can result in headache or even stroke. Malfunctioning nerves in the head may cause pain or paralysis. Glands in the head that produce tears and saliva may become inflamed, blocked up, or even give rise to tumors. Figure 12 illustrates areas of pain in the head.

The temporomandibular joint (TMJ), like certain other joints, contains a meniscus or shock absorber made of cartilage. If you have pain involving one or both jaws, particularly when chewing, you may suffer from disease or poor function of the TMJ. A very common problem is the TMJ syndrome where the muscles surrounding the joint have become extremely tense and cause the joint to function improperly. Patients often feel that their jaw grinds, clicks, or perhaps even locks at times.

Alternatively, the TMJ syndrome may be the result of problems within the joint itself, whether from injury or poor occlusion of the teeth either of which can cause the muscles to tense as a secondary response. The resulting chronic pain in the jaw can move to the ear or the neck. Pain is particularly worse in the morning because patients tend to clench their teeth at night. TMJ syndrome may also be responsible for certain cases of neck pain, migraine, or chronic tension headache.

The temporomandibular joint may also be affected by *rheumatoid arthritis*. A patient suffering from rheumatoid arthritis of the jaw may describe pain or stiffness in jaw movement after periods of jaw inactivity. This stiffness may alleviate somewhat with continued motion of the jaw.

If you experience severe forehead pain, scalp tenderness, or headache, you may be suffering from *temporal arteritis,* also known as *giant cell arteritis.* With this disease, blood vessels in the scalp, jaw, tongue, and the eye become inflamed, decreasing the blood flow to these areas. Indeed, many areas of the body may be affected by temporal arteritis. In the region of the head, you may experience pain in one or both sides of the jaw while chewing. You may also feel pain in the ear, tongue, throat, or even the back of the head. You may experience fatigue, fever, weight loss, or simply "feel ill."

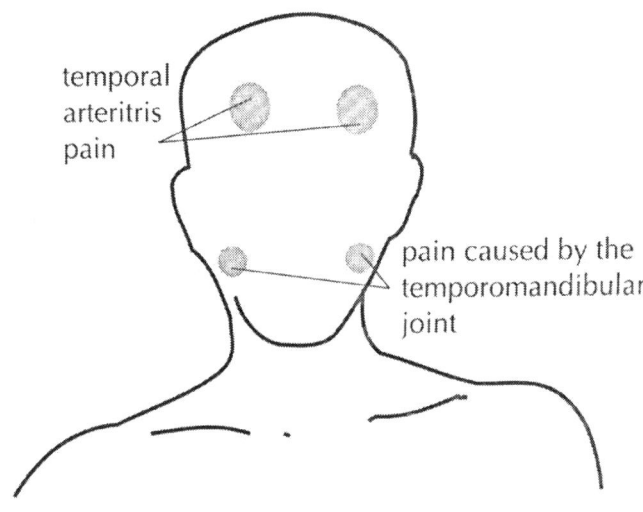

temporal arteritris pain

pain caused by the temporomandibular joint

Figure 12. Areas of pain in the head.

Most often, this disease strikes people over 50. It can start suddenly or very slowly. If the artery on the forehead is tender or enlarged, this may be an early warning of the disease.

Temporal arteritis is associated with *polymyalgia rheumatica,* occurring in about twenty percent of patients with temporal arteritis.

The greatest hazard of temporal arteritis is the possibility of sudden and permanent blindness in one or both eyes if it affects the blood vessels leading to the eye. Heart attacks and strokes have also been linked with temporal arteritis, albeit very rarely. Though it can be catastrophic, temporal arteritis is treatable and often curable if diagnosed and treated promptly.

A *migraine headache,* also called a *vascular headache,* is a most severe type of headache. The onset of a migraine is often preceded by a sensorial aura in which the blood vessels in the head start to constrict. When the blood vessels enlarge, the migraine headache occurs. There are several types of migraine headache, many of which are accompanied by nausea, vomiting, and the inability to look at light. Some people describe seeing flashing lights. Nowadays, migraines are quite preventable and treatable in most patients.

If tightness in the neck precedes your headaches, you may be suffering from *muscle tension headache.* This occurs when the neck muscles tighten up, sometimes in response to excess stress. The muscle tightness spreads to the temples and the scalp as well as the forehead; some patients describe it as feeling like "a band around the head." Tension headaches can be so severe that they induce nausea and vomiting. They can also be associated with migraine headaches.

Sinus headaches occur when the sinuses drain poorly and allow excess mucus and infected material to accumulate. Patients often describe stuffy, tender cheeks or foreheads. Fortunately, sinus headaches are almost always treatable.

If you suffer from severe, piercing pain on only one side of your face, it may be the result of nerve disease. *Tic douloureux* or *trigeminal neuralgia* is an episodic sharp pain of unclear cause that occurs repeatedly. Shingles or herpes zoster may produce similar facial pain after infection and the telltale skin rash. The pain can be sharp and chronic. Both types of facial pain, while quite disabling, are very often treatable.

If the above causes do not explain the pain in your face and head, the

83

origins of the problems may be elsewhere. Angina (diminished blood flow in heart blood vessels), often felt as chest pressure, is transmitted to the jaw. At times, though, angina may be felt only in the jaw. When jaw pain occurs with exertion, this may be a clue to poor blood flow to the heart.

Another possible cause of facial pain may be found in the parotid gland. Located at the jaw immediately in front of the ear, the parotid gland usually swells when it becomes painful. It may become infected or swell because of a blocked duct from the gland. Ingested or injected iodine can sometimes cause the gland to inflame, as can certain viruses. In *Sjögren's syndrome,* the gland may become inflamed because of an underlying connective tissue disease. Finally, certain tumors may arise from and cause pain in the parotid gland.

Facial pain of any kind warrants a very careful evaluation, because most causes of facial pain are treatable and certain types of facial pain may be an outward sign of a more serious underlying condition.

Hoarseness may also warrant a thorough search for an underlying cause. Aside from throat problems, hoarseness may suggest other underlying conditions, such as esophagus difficulties tumor, heart disease, rheumatoid arthritis, or an underactive thyroid gland *(hypothyroid).*

The Neck

The bone structure of the neck is very similar to that of the low back. The basic building blocks are the vertebral bodies, which are separated by the shock-absorbing discs of cartilage. The vertebral bodies are joined in the back of the neck at each level by two facet joints. The spinal cord travels through the spinal canal, emitting nerve roots at each level. These nerve roots, in turn, lead to the more peripheral nerves traveling out from the spinal cord. Figure 13 shows the areas of pain at the back of the neck.

The complicated structure of the neck makes it vulnerable to a wide variety of problems. A herniated *(ruptured) disc* or a *bony spur* in the neck can press on one of the nerve roots, causing a radiating pain that reaches down the shoulder into the arm. This can be felt as numbness, tingling, burning, and/or weakness. A ruptured disc in the neck may occur spontaneously, especially if the disc has been previously injured or diseased. Disc rupture may also occur with trauma, such as "whiplash," in a car accident, and may be associated with neck *muscle strain.* Likewise, a *neck ligament sprain* may occur after such an injury. Remember, a *strain* occurs when a muscle is overstretched and sometimes tears; a *sprain* is when a ligament develops a tear.

If you develop pain in your neck after holding it in an unusual position (such as cradling a phone against your ear) or after exposure to cold, you may be suffering from *wryneck*—a simple neck muscle spasm. This may be part of a generalized *fibromyalgia* syndrome in which tender points develop in the muscles of the neck as well as in other muscular areas of the body, such as the back. Neck tightness and muscle spasms, accompanied by a tension headache, are generally attributable to stress and a lack of quality sleep.

Neck pain may also be the result of *osteoarthritis.* Most people over the age of 50 will have experienced some osteoarthritic changes; however, these changes do not always lead to neck pain. Certainly, severe osteoarthritis affecting the facet joint can cause neck pain, as well as bony spurs which may press on nerve roots in the spine and lead to pain radiating into the shoulder and arm.

Rheumatoid arthritis is less common than osteoarthritis in the neck region. However, rheumatoid arthritis may affect the upper neck and loosen the supporting tissues at the very top of the spine. It is important to check for the loosening of these tissues in patients who have rheumatoid arthritis, particularly in preparation for surgery. During general anesthesia induction, the head may be tilted back and the spinal cord compressed by loose bone in the neck, which can result in permanent paralysis below the neck.

Enthesopathy, particularly *ankylosing spondylitis,* may also involve the

85

neck. While this may cause just pain and stiffness initially, it can eventually cause a rigid neck fixed in one position if ankylosis or bony fusing of the neck occurs.

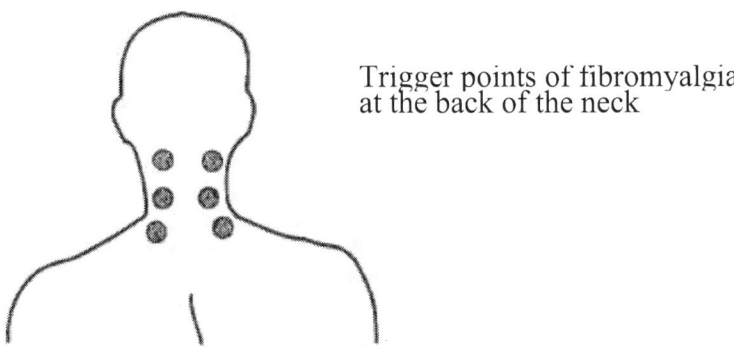

Trigger points of fibromyalgia at the back of the neck

Figure 13. Areas of pain at the back of the neck

If your neck pain coincides with muscle ache elsewhere in the body, you may be suffering from one of a number of different diseases. *Fibromyalgia,* which can involve the thighs and the entire back, also can cause aching and stiffness in the neck. *Polymyalgia rheumatica* is a low-grade inflammatory condition of the muscles, often involving the thighs, calves, upper arms, shoulders and back, as well as the neck. You might feel stiffness, particularly upon waking in the morning, in any or all of these parts of your body.

There are several causes of *myopathy* (a general term for muscle disease) in the neck, simply because the neck involves such a mass of muscle. One of these diseases is *myositis,* a severe inflammatory condition of the large muscles. If you experience neck weakness, perhaps with neck pain, the problem may be myositis, which can lead to muscle destruction.

Migraine headaches are often associated with neck pain, and on occasion, may be located primarily in the neck. Migraines are also associated with tension headaches which often find their origins in the muscles in the back of the neck.

If the pain in your neck feels connected to your jaw, you may be suffering from *temporomandibular joint* or *TMJ syndrome.* With this ailment, you can experience pain on one or both sides of the jaw while chewing. The increased tension developed in the chewing muscles may spread into neck muscles, resulting in neck pain.

If you are experiencing pain in the front of the neck, the problem may stem from *thyroiditis,* an inflammation of the thyroid gland. This inflammation is often the result of autoantibodies becoming misprogrammed to attack one's own thyroid gland. Tumors of the thyroid may also cause pain in the front of the neck.

Enlargement of the lymph nodes accompanying a variety of infections may cause pain in either the front or the back of the neck. An infection is usually readily apparent, but occasionally its location and exact cause remain obscure.

Finally, pain can sometimes travel to the neck from the shoulder or even the wrist as with *carpal tunnel syndrome*. In this syndrome, compression of the median nerve at the wrist occurs from any of several different causes. The pain produced may travel back up the arm occasionally as high as the shoulder and neck. In this situation, it appears as if a nerve root is being compressed in the neck, causing pain to travel down the arm but, in fact, it is actually the reverse. Treatment is directed at the source in the wrist.

The Shoulder

The shoulder is a very complicated and mobile joint. It is actually composed of four joints, collectively called the shoulder girdle. Over the top of the shoulder, the rotator cuff is formed by four tendons, enabling the upper arm to move in a variety of directions. Because

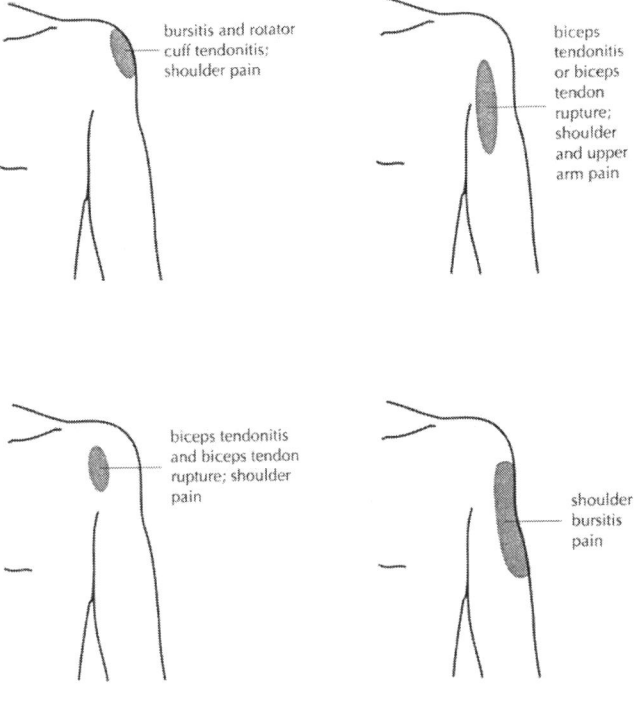

Figure 14. Areas of pain in the shoulder.

of its complexity and mobility, the shoulder is not very stable, and so it is subject to a large number of problems. Figure 14 shows areas of pain in the shoulder.

If you have pain, weakness, or difficulty in raising your arm from your side (outward and upward, like the hand of a clock), you may be suffering from *rotator cuff disease* or a *shoulder bursitis. Rotator cuff tendinopathy* often occurs with bursitis and vice versa. Both cause tenderness and weakness in the upper outer shoulder, and pain when you lift the arm as described above, or attempt to sleep in bed. Rotator cuff tendinopathy may be caused by the CORE diseases or by the presence of bony spurs pressing on the tendon. When a spur presses on the rotator cuff as you lift your arm, you are experiencing what is called the *impingement syndrome.* A complete tear of the rotator cuff makes it very difficult for you to lift your arm upward and outward. Partial rotator cuff tears, once thought to be the exclusive domain of baseball pitchers, occur fairly frequently in people older than 45. The daily traumatic stress of work and play coupled with degenerative change of the tendon makes this problem commonplace.

The shoulder joints themselves may be affected by various types of arthritis, especially the CORE diseases. In addition, the shoulder joints may become infected with bacteria or other infectious organisms. *Hemochromatosis* or iron overload disease may also involve the shoulder.

Osteoarthritis involving the joint between the humerus (upper arm bone) and the shoulder blade can cause both pain as well as limited range of motion. When the arthritis has progressed to this degree, shoulder replacement surgery may need to be considered.

If you have difficulty in moving your shoulder, you may also be suffering from *frozen shoulder,* also called *adhesive capsulitis.* Along with restricted movement, you may feel extreme pain even with the slightest gesture. Pain occurs particularly in bed at night. Any affliction of the shoulder may bring on this condition. The frozen shoulder occurs as a result of the limitation of movement in the shoulder. For unclear reasons, the shoulder capsule becomes thickened, resulting in frozen shoulder, which still further restricts shoulder mobility.

It is sometimes difficult to discover the original cause of the condition if you have been suffering with it for a long time. Very often, treating the frozen shoulder is more difficult than treating the underlying problem.

Shoulder stiffness and pain in particular may be associated with *polymyalgia rheumatica, diabetes mellitus,* and *hyperthyroidism* (overactive thyroid).

The biceps tendon, located in the front of the shoulder, may be a source of your shoulder pain. When this tendon moves in and out of its groove, it is called a *subluxed bicep tendon* and feels as if the shoulder is popping in and out of place. The bicep tendon may become inflamed by any one of the CORE diseases as well as by bony spurs and excessive use *(biceps tendinopathy).* This tendon may even tear, causing the biceps muscle to form into a ball on the front of the upper arm. This looks like a muscle on a muscle or what we call *Popeye's sign* of a *biceps tendon rupture.*

Aseptic necrosis may cause severe destructive change at the top of the upper arm, leading to severe shoulder pain. This is often associated with a history of chronic cortisone (steroid) use. For reasons that are not yet clear, cortisone compromises the blood supply, leading to dead and crumbling bone.

The *shoulder-hand syndrome* or the *reflex sympathetic dystrophy syndrome (RSD)* or *chronic regional pain syndrome (CRPS)* is a poorly understood problem in which the shoulder becomes stiff and loses movement and the hand becomes swollen and painful. The hand may feel hot or cold. Injury to the shoulder, periods of immobility following a stroke or heart attack, surgery, and certain drugs such as barbiturates and isoniazid may bring on this condition. Eventually, you can lose the use of the hand and the shoulder if the syndrome continues.

Excruciating shoulder pain may originate in areas outside the shoulder. The *carpal tunnel syndrome,* described above, may cause pain to shoot up the arm into the shoulder. Nerve root irritation in the neck may similarly cause pain to travel down the neck and into the shoulder.

Even ailments in the torso may affect the shoulder. Tumors in the chest may cause pain to radiate to the shoulder. Abdominal diseases, including those affecting the gallbladder and liver, as well as pleurisy may transmit pain to the tip of the shoulder blade.

A nerve root may become pinched by a *bony spur* or a *ruptured (herniated) disc* as it exits the spinal cord in the neck. This may cause pain, weakness, tingling, burning, or numbness on the affected side in the shoulder, arm, and head.

After nerve roots exit from the spinal cord in the neck, they form the *brachial plexus,* an arrangement of nerves from which the more peripheral nerves travel down the arm. The collar bone or neck muscles may press on the brachial plexus, causing pain to shoot into the shoulder as well as the arms and the hand. Numbness, tingling, and burning may also occur. This is called *thoracic outlet syndrome.*

The brachial plexus may also be affected by *diabetes,* injuries to the area, tumor, infection, or radiation used to treat tumors, resulting in significant pain to the shoulder and the arm.

Shoulder tumors (either directly arising in the bone or travelling from remote sites) may cause severe shoulder pain. *Fibromyalgia,* discussed elsewhere, may attack the muscle areas surrounding the shoulder and overlying the shoulder blade, provoking muscle tightness and spasm, and causing pain to travel into the shoulder and down the arm.

Lastly, *angina,* or poor blood flow in the arteries of the heart may produce pain in the left shoulder, particularly with exercise.

The Upper Arm

The upper arm, lying between the shoulder and the elbow, is the site of attachment of substantial muscles, including the biceps, triceps, and deltoid. It also functions as a conduit through which the blood vessels and nerves reach the forearm and hand. Figure 15 shows areas of pain in the upper arm.

Many causes of upper arm pain are identical to the causes of shoulder pain described below. *Shoulder bursitis, biceps tendinopathy* or even *biceps tendon rupture* can affect the upper arm. The last is often accompanied by sudden pain and a curling of the biceps muscle into a small lump that protrudes over the front of the upper arm.

Pain, tingling, weakness, and/or numbness may occur due to pressure on nerve roots or on the nerves themselves as described above with a *ruptured (herniated) disc* in the neck, the *thoracic outlet syndrome,* or in *brachial plexus* injuries.

Because the upper arm has a fairly sizable muscle mass, it is subject to the various diseases that can affect the muscle. *Polymyalgia rheumatica, myositis,* and *fibromyalgia,* all discussed elsewhere, may strike the upper arm.

Pain from outside the area, such as a pinched nerve in the neck, may course down through the upper arm. Similarly, *carpal tunnel syndrome* may cause pain to travel upward from the wrist through the forearm and the upper arm and beyond to the shoulder and even the neck.

Knowing whether the pain is located on one side or both sides is helpful in determining the cause of upper arm pain. *Polymyalgia rheumatica, myositis,* and other muscle diseases are systemic—that is, they tend to occur in both upper arms at the same time. All the other conditions described above usually occur or at least start on one side. Angina, for example, poor blood flow to the heart, may produce pain and/or numbness in the left upper arm.

The Elbow

The elbow is the joint where the upper arm and forearm meet. It is the junction of three bones (two from the forearm, one from the upper arm) into three joints. This complex structure permits bending and straightening of the upper arm in relation to the forearm as well as rotating the forearm and hand. Figure 16 shows areas of discomfort of the elbows.

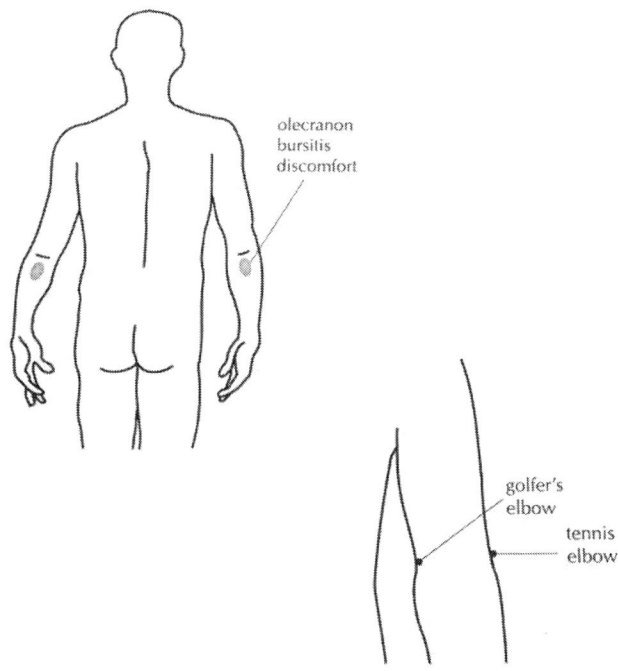

Figure 16. Areas of pain in the elbow

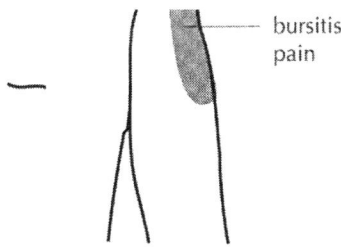

Figure 15. Areas of pain in the upper arm.

Elbow pain may originate from directly within the elbow or from areas surrounding the elbow. The CORE diseases may involve the elbow joints directly. In addition, the elbow may become infected with *bacteria* or other organisms, causing pain with any movement of the elbow and leaving it red, hot, tender, and swollen. *Sarcoidosis* may also inflame the elbow. The most comfortable (or the least uncomfortable) position in such cases is keeping the elbow slightly bent. When the elbow is completely straightened or completely bent, the volume of the joint decreases, which increases pressure within the elbow as well as the pain.

If you experience a large, almost rubbery swelling at the end of the elbow, you may have an *olecranon bursitis.* This condition may result from repeated injury caused by leaning on the elbow. This bursitis may also be associated with infection, *crystal diseases,* and *rheumatoid arthritis.* Because this bursa does not connect directly to the elbow, movement is usually painless and completely normal.

If shaking hands, lifting a briefcase, or flicking your knuckles back towards the wrist causes pain in the elbow, you may have what is called *tennis elbow.* Most people who develop this do not play tennis; it is simply a tendinopathy on the outside aspect of the elbow. *Golfer's elbow* is tendinopathy on the inside aspect of the elbow and is much less common than tennis elbow.

If you experience aching on the inner aspect of the elbow and tenderness near your "funny bone" you may be suffering from problems with the ulnar nerve. This nerve moves down the inside of the forearm to the small finger and the side of the ring finger facing the small finger. You may feel numbness or tingling in these fingers, particularly if you lift your hand to your head. You may also become clumsy with the affected hand. This problem is generally the result of *ulnar nerve entrapment* from keeping your elbows on the arms of an armchair, for example, or from an injury or fracture in that area. Chronic misuse in certain occupations, in which the inner elbow is subject to repeated pressure and/or trauma, may also cause this condition.

The Forearm

The forearm consists of two parallel bones between the wrist and the elbow. It serves as an anchor for the muscles and tendons which allow for the remarkable dexterity of the fingers. As described above, pain experienced on the inner aspect of the forearm on the side of the small finger may be due to disease or pressure on the ulnar nerve. This is often accompanied by tingling, numbness, pain, and/or weakness in the small finger and the aspect of the ring finger facing it. *Ulnar nerve compression* may occur at either the wrist or the elbow. Figure 17 illustrates areas of pain in the forearm.

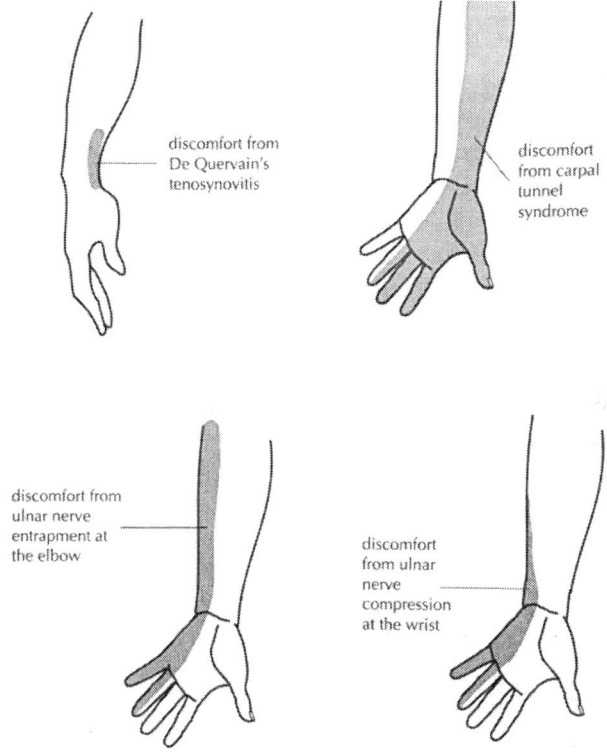

discomfort from De Quervain's tenosynovitis

discomfort from carpal tunnel syndrome

discomfort from ulnar nerve entrapment at the elbow

discomfort from ulnar nerve compression at the wrist

Figure 17. Areas of pain in the forearm.

Similarly, *carpal tunnel syndrome* is the result of compression on the median nerve at the wrist. This nerve, going to the first four fingers of the hand (starting with the thumb), travels through the wrist, the forearm, the upper arm, and into the shoulder and neck. Pain from this nerve may shoot up the arm, sometimes reaching the shoulder and the neck. People suffering from carpal tunnel syndrome may experience numbness, tingling, or a sharp or dull pain, particularly upon waking up in the morning.

Pain, arm weakness, tingling, and/or numbness may be due to a pinched nerve or nerve root in or near the neck. This can occur with a *herniated (ruptured) disc, thoracic outlet syndrome,* or *brachial plexus* injury.

Another cause of pain in the forearm is *tendinopathy* affecting the tendons controlling the hand and fingers. This is a fairly common affliction after overuse. When it affects the tendon involving the thumb, it is called *Dequervains tenosynovitis.* You can determine if you have tendinopathy by bending your thumb into the palm of your hand and closing the fingers over it in a fist. If this gesture causes pain,

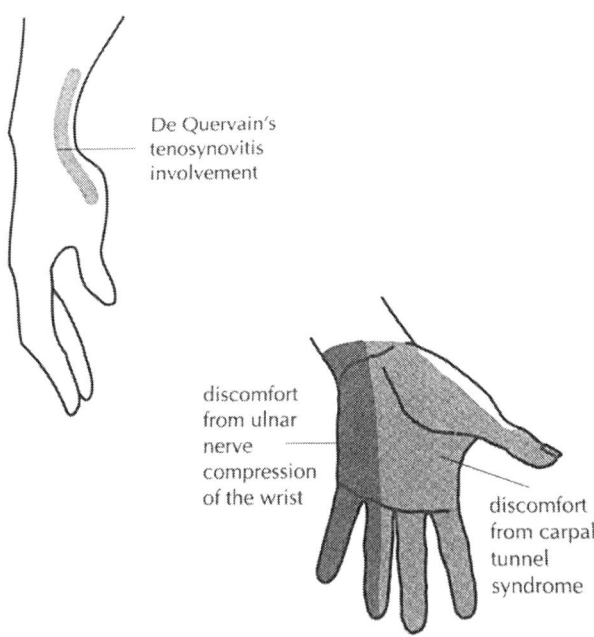

Figure 18. Areas of pain in the wrist and hand.

particularly in the thumb and partway up the forearm, then you probably have tendinopathy.

Angina, poor circulation within the heart, may also cause pain or numbness to radiate down into the left forearm.

The Wrist

The wrist consists of eight small bones forming a hinge with the ends of the two long bones of the forearm. Its purposes are to establish a base for the slender hand bones and protect the vital nerves, blood vessels, and tendons to the fingers. The wrist also enables us to position our hands and fingers in numerous positions, making them so useful in such a wide variety of different ways. Figure 18 shows areas of pain in the wrist and hand.

Pain directly involving the wrist joint may occur from the CORE diseases or from *bacterial infections* (including *gonorrhea)* as well as *Lyme disease* and *tuberculosis. Sarcoidosis* may also involve the wrist. *Hemochromatosis,* iron overload disease, is yet another condition that can affect the wrist.

The tendons in the wrist act as pulleys to move the fingers in the hand. With inflamed wrist tendons, it is difficult to move the wrist by yourself because of the pain. Overuse of the affected wrist and hand may cause tendon inflammation, but this may also result from the CORE diseases. When the wrist is directly affected by arthritis, any movement—by yourself or anyone else—is painful.

Nerve entrapment can occur at the wrist. The median nerve is involved with the thumb and first three fingers of the hand. If this nerve is compressed, you may experience numbness, tingling, burning, and/or weakness in these fingers. *Carpal tunnel syndrome,* discussed in further detail elsewhere, has its origins in the wrist. Similarly, the ulnar nerve, which also passes through the wrist, can be compressed at the wrist, causing numbness, tingling, burning, and/or weakness in the small finger and the facing side of the ring finger *(ulnar nerve compression).* These ailments often result from occupational use and abuse, such as using a jackhammer or resting your wrists against the edge of a desk or table for extended periods of time. It may also occur when arthritis inflames the wrist and presses directly on these nerves.

If you notice a lump or swelling on the top of your wrist, you may have a *ganglion cyst.* This is usually a painless swelling which is full of thick fluid. The ganglion often connects with the wrist or a tendon sheath. Usually, no treatment is required because the ganglion typically causes no pain, poses no threat to the tendon, and may disappear on its own.

Experiencing pain and tenderness over the wrist on the thumb side may be due to *Dequervains tenosynovitis,* and inflammation of the tendons which moves the thumb. When you make a fist over your thumb, your pain will increase with this condition. This is usually the result of excessive repetitive movement of the thumb.

If you simply wake up one day with a flaccid wrist, you may be experiencing *radial nerve palsy.* Also called "bridegroom palsy," this ailment is caused by the compression of the radial nerve at the elbow. Another name for this problem is "Saturday night palsy," so called because if you lean your arm over the back of a chair for a prolonged period of time, you can press on the radial nerve at the elbow.

The Hand

The structure of the hand is best understood in terms of its main function—dexterity of movement and sensation. The fingers are composed of narrow bones hinged together. Delicate tendons allow for movement of each individual finger, while the fingertips are loaded with tiny nerve endings to help serve as our chief instrument in our sense of touch Figure 19 shows areas of pain in the hand.

If you feel pain bending your thumb, the problem lies in one of several areas. *Osteoarthritis* may affect the thumb, particularly at the base, where it will produce a firm yet sensitive bony enlargement. Pain on the top of thumb, which increases when you hold your thumb against your palm and wrap the fingers around it in a fist, may be the result of *Dequervains tenosynovitis.* This is a thumb tendonitis that can extend pain up to the wrist and even into the forearm. Making a fist with the affected hands is one test to determine if the condition is present.

Another form of tendonitis might be indicated when you bend your thumb. Along the tendon that runs at the bottom of the thumb, a small nodule may form, causing the thumb to lock when you try to straighten it.

Stiffness of the hands may be the result of *rheumatoid arthritis and other connective tissue diseases,* particularly *scleroderma* and *lupus. Diabetes mellitus* as well as scleroderma may cause hand stiffness as well as thickening of the skin of the fingers.

Numbness, tingling, or burning in any of the first four fingers (starting with the thumb), which occurs particularly at night or in the morning may be due to *carpal tunnel syndrome.* This occurs when the medial nerve becomes compressed as it passes through the wrist. The carpal tunnel is actually a tunnel made up of bones and ligaments through which the median nerve passes, extending to the first four fingers. This ailment may stem from excessive use, arthritic inflammation or even infection such as *tuberculosis* with the wrist.

Tumors within the wrist, swelling due to pregnancy or low thyroid hormone levels may also provide the cause. *Diabetes* too may affect the median nerve, causing symptoms similar to those found with carpal tunnel syndrome. With carpal tunnel syndrome, your handshake is weak and clumsy, and the pain may move retrograde up the forearm from the fingers toward the shoulder or even the neck. The pain tends to be worse in the morning because fluids accumulate in the wrist with lack of movement and many of us tend to bend the wrist when we sleep.

Likewise, numbness, tingling, or burning in the ring finger and small finger may be caused by disease or compression of the ulnar nerve at the wrist. This may be caused by many of the same factors that cause *carpal tunnel syndrome* (see above).

Pain, tingling, numbness, burning, or weakness may be a result of irritated nerves at or near the neck. Such is the case, for example, with a *herniated (ruptured) disc* in the neck, the *thoracic outlet syndrome,* and *brachial plexus* injury.

Tendonitis may lead to pain and swelling on the palm or on the top of the entire hand. The CORE diseases as well as *sarcoidosis, gonorrhea,* and other infections may inflame the tendons in the hand, though the most common cause of tendonitis is excessive use. The fingers may partially lock or "trigger"—that is, you exert the muscle until the tendon snaps the finger into position—and small tendon nodules may appear, particularly on the palm and the finger.

There are three types of joints in the fingers. These include the knuckles (the *metacarpal phalangeal joints)* where the fingers join the palm, the middle joints (the *proximal interphalangeal joints),* and the joints near the ends of the fingers (the *distal interphalangeal joints).* All of these may be affected by various forms of arthritis, though *osteoarthritis* generally affects only the proximal and the distal interphalangeal joints in the fingers.

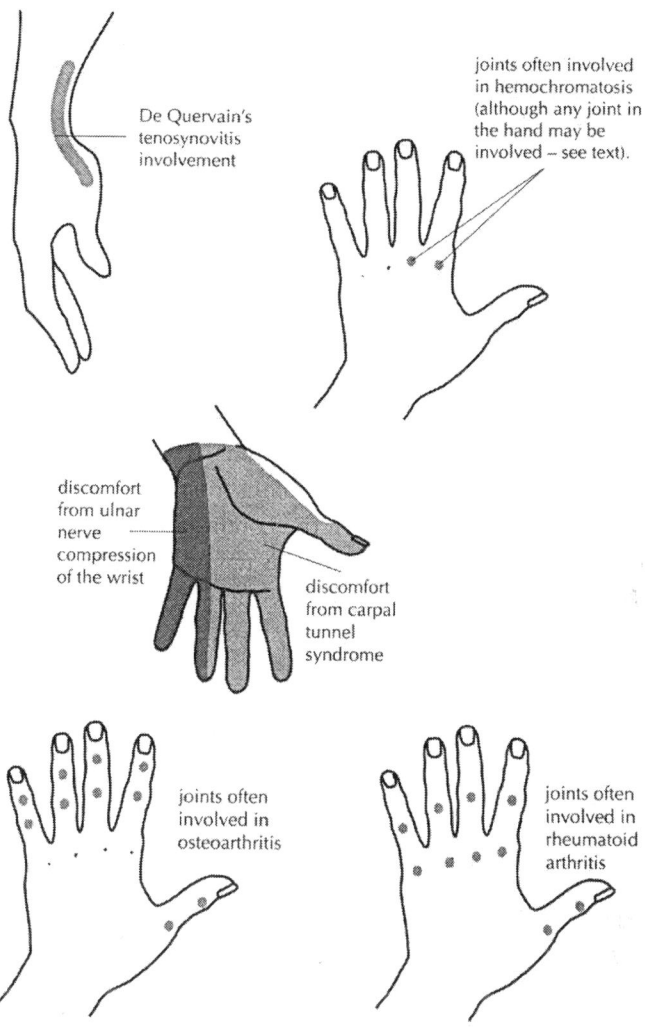

Figure 19. Areas of pain in the hand.

When osteoarthritis affects these joints, it forms bony knobs, causing the fingers to turn in one direction or another. *Rheumatoid arthritis* and *connective tissue diseases,* on the other hand, may strike the metacarpal and proximal interphalangeal joints, causing the knuckles and middle joints to be stiff for at least an hour in the morning. The *crystal diseases* and *enthesopathies* may also involve the finger joints, as can *hyperlipidemia* (elevated blood cholesterol or triglycerides), *Lyme disease,* and *sarcoidosis.*

Another disease, *hemochromatosis,* can involve the knuckles. In this disease, the gastrointestinal system absorbs too much iron, causing the joints to swell and inflame. This can also cause stiffness, particularly of the knuckles of the index and middle fingers, but may involve any joint in the hand.

If your hands are constantly cold, you may be suffering from *Raynaud's phenomenon.* This is associated with various *connective tissue diseases* and leads to changes in the color of the hands when they are exposed to cold air or water. The fingers may turn in succession white, blue, then red. This condition is due to an extreme sensitivity to the cold, which causes the small arteries in the fingers to constrict excessively.

Raynaud's phenomenon is generally associated with *connective tissue disease,* but it also may be a side effect of certain medications, especially ergots (used for treating migraines) and beta-blockers (used for heart disease and high blood pressure). There are even occasions where there is no particular underlying disease whatsoever, in which case the condition is diagnosed as *Raynaud's disease.*

Another cause of coldness in the hand is *shoulder-hand syndrome* or *reflex sympathetic dystrophy syndrome* or *chronic regional pain syndrome,* often as a result of an injury to the shoulder or some other condition that has left the shoulder immobilized. This is described in greater detail in the section on the shoulder.

Tingling or numbness in the hand may be the result of a *peripheral neuropathy. A peripheral neuropathy* occurs when the nerves in the skin misfire, causing you to feel such sensations as burning or tingling even when the stimuli for such sensations are not present. Peripheral neuropathy involving the entire hand is often associated with numerous diseases and medicinal side effects. This involvement of the entire hand is in contrast to both *carpal tunnel syndrome,* which affects the first four fingers of the hand (starting with the thumb) and *ulnar nerve compression,* which usually affects the small finger and the adjacent side of the ring finger.

Among the diseases associated with peripheral neuropathy in the entire hand are *diabetes mellitus, tumors, connective tissue diseases* (including *lupus, rheumatoid arthritis, scleroderma, mixed connective tissue disorder, overlap syndrome,* and *Sjögren's syndrome), thyroid disease, Lyme disease, alcohol abuse, leprosy,* and a variety of *vitamin deficiencies.*

There are also certain medications and a variety of chemicals associated with peripheral neuropathy. Among drugs and medications that cause as a side effect peripheral neuropathy are excess vitamin B6 (used for B6 deficiency), hydroxychloroquine (used for the treatment of rheumatoid arthritis and lupus), metronidazole (used for vaginal trichomonas), cisplatin and vincristine (both used in cancer chemotherapy), hydralazine (high blood pressure), isoniazid (tuberculosis), and various others. Arsenic and organophosphates, common chemicals in insecticides, can similarly cause peripheral neuropathy. Finally, alcohol can diminish physical sensitivity and produce numbness as well.

If the last two fingers (the ring and small) of your hand have a marked propensity to bend in unison toward the palm, you may be experiencing *Dupuytren's contracture.* This is a painless condition resulting from the thickening of the tissue in the palm that usually involves the ring finger. Occurring more frequently in men than women, it is benign, but may be associated with such conditions as chronic alcohol use and epilepsy.

If your hand swells, it can be the outcome of any one of a number of problems. *Shoulder-hand syndrome* (also called *reflex sympathetic dystrophy syndrome* or *chronic regional pain syndrome)* which, as we saw, can leave your hands feeling cold, may also cause the entire hand to swell. Such inflammatory diseases as the *crystal diseases, rheumatoid arthritis,* the *connective tissue diseases,* and the *enthesopathies* may cause the joints and tendons of the hand to swell. In these cases, the patient's hands are stiff and feel as if they are wearing gloves. Such bacterial infections as *gonorrhea* may cause similar swelling. The use of certain medications (such as quinidine) or the general lack of use of the hand can lead to diffuse swelling. This is particularly true of stroke victims, who may find that the hand they do not use becomes swollen and stiff. Finally, an overactive thyroid gland *(hyperthyroid)* may cause diffuse swelling of the hands, a condition termed *thyroid acropachy.*

The Chest

The chest is designed for both movement and protection. The ribs, for example, serve as a movable frame, allowing for expansion and contraction of the chest wall as we breathe. The bony ribs are able to move only because they are connected to the breastbone (the sternum) by soft pliable cartilage. The ribs form a protective cage for the heart and lungs. A layer of muscle covers the ribs completely, adding another measure of protection for the individual. Most of the larger muscles in the chest help to move the shoulder. The muscular diaphragm forms the bottom of the chest cavity and enables us to breathe. Figure 20 shows areas of pain in the chest.

Since chest pain can be a very ominous symptom, most people wisely have their doctor evaluate the problem immediately. A great deal of the time, however, such pain is not the result of heart or lung disease.

If you experience pain in the region of the breast bone, it may be originating in the chest wall cartilage. This occurs at the costochondral junction, where the cartilage connects the ribs to the breast bone. When the cartilage becomes inflamed, a condition also termed *Tietzes's syndrome* or *costochondritis,* it causes sharp pain in the upper chest that may radiate to the shoulder or arm. The pain worsens when you take a deep breath, sneeze, cough, or bend, or directly touch the area.

Pain at the tip of the sternum is called *sternal tip syndrome.* Sometimes the result of injury or trauma, sometimes the outcome of an unclear cause, this feeling can be reproduced somewhat by pressing on the tip of the breast bone. It may result in nausea, vomiting, or pain in the pit of the stomach.

Nearly any rib may be at the source of chest pain. For example, the lower ribs can cause significant chest pain in a patient who develops a hunched back *(kyphosis)* following a compression fracture of the upper spine. Such fractures often occur from *osteoporosis* and cause a very sharp pain which shoots from the upper back along both sides of the chest.

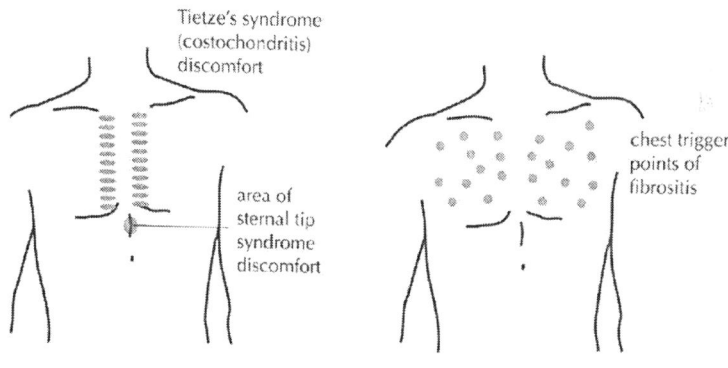

Figure 20. Areas of pain in the chest.

Nearly any area of the chest may be involved by *fibromyalgia*, a condition affecting the soft tissues. Sometimes the older name *fibrositis* is seen in the literature. Small tender areas, called trigger points, develop in many areas of the chest. Although they are exquisitely tender, these trigger points usually respond well to treatment.

Other causes of chest pain may be rib fractures or the manifestations of the early onset of *shingles.* Shingles, caused by the same virus that causes chicken pox, resides in the spinal nerve roots. It may show itself at times by a red rash comprised of small blisters that seem to follow a line along one side of the body. Before the appearance of the rash, you may feel severe or burning pain on one side of your back or on the outside or front of your chest.

The gastrointestinal tract is a fairly common source of chest discomfort. Acid may reflux—that is, move up from the stomach through the esophagus to the mouth. When this occurs, you may experience heartburn and taste the contents of the stomach. The reflux of acid may also cause you to drool, particularly when you sleep, so you may find a saliva residue on the pillow when you wake up.

Acid reflux may cause not only cause hoarseness; it may cause spasms of the esophagus, the muscular tube that connects the mouth to the stomach. When this happens, you may feel severe chest pain and tenderness in the chest wall itself. Nitroglycerin may stop the esophagus spasm, thereby relieving the chest pain.

Though nitroglycerin will affect reflux-induced chest pain, the fact that it works will not help specify the cause of the pain. Reflux remains poorly understood. To complicate matters, many connective tissue diseases can lead a patient to develop a propensity for gastroesophageal reflux. With or without connective tissue disease, if there is relaxation of the usually taut muscles at the end of the esophagus near the stomach, reflux may occur.

Whatever the cause, gastroesophageal reflux is an underappreciated and common cause of chest pain in the general population.

Angina, poor blood flow to the heart muscle, usually produces a feeling of chest pressure or "squeezing" behind the breastbone. This may be accompanied by nausea, shortness of breath, and excess sweating. The pain may move to the neck or jaw or even down the arm (usually the left arm).

Pericarditis is inflammation of the outside lining of the heart. The pain is a sharp, stabbing one that increases with deep breathing. The pain is located behind the breastbone or slightly to the left of it.

Pleurisy is inflammation of the lining of the lung. The pain is sharp and increases upon taking a deep breath. The pain may be located in any portion of the front or back of the chest. Unlike many other conditions affecting the chest, pleurisy does not leave the chest tender to touch.

Finally, *tumors* may cause quite severe chest pain. Such tumors may arise from sites outside the ribs and migrate or metastasize to the bony ribs. *Breast cancer* and *lung cancer* are two such tumors that behave in this fashion.

People with muscle disease complain of pain, stiffness, cramps, and/or weakness in the large muscle groups such as the thighs, calves, upper arms, neck, and low back. The muscles may hurt *(myalgias),* be inflamed *(myositis),* or simply be weak *(myasthenia).*

The most important distinction to mark here is that between *weakness* and *fatigue. Weakness* is the lack of strength; *fatigue* is the lack of energy. Unfortunately, many people use one term when they really mean the other. Of course, weakness may accompany fatigue. What complicates the matter is that when you experience pain in a particular region of the body, you will not forcibly move that area. It makes perfectly good sense, of course, but it may result in a false impression of weakness.

It sometimes takes a great deal of patience and perseverance to identify specific muscle disease. Such efforts are often rewarded, however, because many muscle conditions are quite treatable.

Muscle Cramps

A muscle cramp, also called a charley horse, is a painful, uncontrolled muscle spasm in which the muscle knots up. Muscle cramps usually occur at rest, particularly at night, and typically involve the calf or the small muscles of the feet.

A number of conditions may predispose you to muscle cramping. Overuse of the muscles, particularly in an unaccustomed activity, may help precipitate the episode. A number of medications may also promote muscle cramping, including clofibrate, danazol, hydralazine, zidovudine, rifampin, carbamazepine, penicillamine, albuterol and terbutaline. Alcohol abuse may also provoke a tendency toward muscle cramping.

Another cause of cramping muscles is a phenomenon called *electrolyte abnormalities,* often the result of a mineral imbalance in the system. Low sodium, magnesium, potassium, and calcium as well as elevated potassium may precipitate cramping. Similarly, certain medications such as diuretics may lead to electrolyte abnormalities.

Still other conditions can lead to muscle cramping. The lowering of blood sugar to very low levels and thyroid disease (both *hyperthyroidism* and *hypothyroidism)* may predispose an individual to muscle cramps. Another situation which commonly causes cramping is exposure to excess heat, which can occur at home, at work, or at play. And patients undergoing kidney dialysis have a tendency to develop muscle cramps.

A final cause of this condition is neurologic. *Lou Gehrig's disease* or *amyotrophic lateral sclerosis (ALS)* is a condition of neurologic deterioration of certain cells in the spinal cord. One symptom of ALS is muscle cramping.

Various general treatments have been prescribed for muscle cramps, including the use of vitamin E and quinine. As always, though, the most important first step toward the effective treatment of the condition is to understand what is causing it in the first place.

Polymyalgia Rheumatica

Emily is a 60-year'old woman who woke up one morning with stiff and achy shoulders, upper arms, thighs, and calves. She described herself as feeling as if she had run a marathon the day before. This feeling continued without change for six weeks. She gradually lost her appetite and felt generally tired, miserable, and depressed.

Her physician diagnosed polymyalgia rheumatica after listening to her story and obtaining the necessary laboratory tests. A moderate dose of cortisone provided relief almost overnight. The cortisone was tapered off gradually over the period of a year. Since that time, Emily has not suffered any relapse of the disease.

Polymyalgia rheumatica (PMR) means "multiple aching muscles."

People suffering with this condition develop stiffness and aching in the shoulders, upper arms, thighs, groin, calves, neck, and low back. Both sides of the body are usually involved, though muscle strength is generally unaffected. Stiffness is particularly prominent upon waking, regardless of whether it is after a short nap or a full night's sleep. Joints as well as muscles may be involved, especially in the hands and wrists.

While the cause remains unknown, PMR affects women more than men, with the majority of patients being over age 50. It is a fairly common condition, affecting roughly one person in 20,000 every year. The onset of PMR may be either abrupt or gradual. Patients describe themselves as simply "not feeling well," suffer some weight loss, have low grade temperatures, and experience both depression and fatigue.

PMR may be associated with *temporal arteritis,* a vasculitis or inflammatory disease of the blood vessels affecting primarily small blood vessels of the head and face. Temporal arteritis may lead to blindness if it inflames the blood vessels in the back of the eye. About eighty percent of people with PMR will not go on to develop temporal arteritis; however, roughly 50 percent of people with temporal arteritis have a prior history of PMR.

PMR may also be followed by the development of *rheumatoid arthritis.* It is not clear, however, if these people initially had a case of rheumatoid arthritis that was imitating PMR or had true PMR prior to the onset of rheumatoid arthritis.

A laboratory test called an *erythrocyte sedimentation rate* (ESR) is usually elevated abnormally in PMR. A certain protein in the blood tends to be produced in excess with this disease. However, not every case of PMR will have an accompanying elevated sedimentation rate. Furthermore, muscle biopsies performed on patients with PMR are always normal.

Fortunately, once diagnosed, PMR is very treatable. Moderate doses of cortisone are begun and then gradually tapered off. Response to treatment is usually dramatic. Half the cases are curable with cortisone; the other cases usually have a good response to treatment but patients may not be able to give up the treatment program. In such cases, patients are usually given low maintenance doses of the medication. PMR can last months or even years.

Fibromyalgia

Michelle, *a 36-year-old court reporter,* described stiffness and pain involving her neck and entire back following a motor vehicle accident two years before. The pain in her neck was first thought to be whiplash, but she went on to develop severe aching and stiffness over her entire back. Poor sleep left her exhausted, and she described her hands and feet as "swelling" although no one else, including her physician, could see it. Her work suffered. She found it difficult to concentrate and lean forward over her stenography machine for prolonged periods. Although always tired, she could not sleep at night because her mind was "racing." She had been to several doctors and began to believe that she was a hypochondriac. Frustrated, she sought narcotics from various doctors, but these pain relievers offered only temporary relief.

While browsing through the newspaper, Michelle came across an article in the health section on fibromyalgia. A visit to a physician familiar with the condition confirmed the diagnosis. Treatment began with physical therapy and medications to deepen her sleep. She responded dramatically, with significant improvement in both her pain and her fatigue. Finally, Michelle's self-image improved noticeably when she realized that her pain had indeed been real.

Alternative names for *fibromyalgia* include *fibrositis* and *fibromyositis*. The term stands for "inflammation of fibrous connective tissue," though there is no true inflammation seen in biopsy specimens under the microscope. Connective tissue is supporting tissue of the body, including ligaments, tendons, and muscles.

To the victim of fibromyalgia, it feels as if these soft tissues are inflamed. Fibromyalgia is a syndrome of chronic, recurring, diffuse aching and stiffness, especially of the whole back and neck. It is a very common condition, accounting for as many as one in every ten patients visiting medical clinics. Women develop fibromyalgia more frequently than men. The usual age group is between 20 and 50, but children, teenagers, and many patients over 50 can also suffer from it.

The cause of fibromyalgia is unclear. Microscopically, there is no evidence of abnormalities in the tissues of patients with fibromyalgia.

Fibromyalgia is thought to be due to a chemical imbalance in the brain. The ability to feel and sense is a result of chemical reactions inside the brain. Certain pathways such as dopamine, serotonin, and norepinephrine become disrupted and this can lead to both allodynia (perceiving a normal stimulus to be painful) and hyperpathia (the sensation that a painful stimulus is more painful than it really is.

Along with pain in the upper and lower back and neck, fibromyalgia causes stiffness and discomfort that varies in severity from day to day. The level of discomfort depends upon a variety of conditions, from the weather and physical activity to the individual's threshold of stress. Discomfort improves with massage, flexibility exercises, heat, restful vacation, and control of stress.

Its onset may be either abrupt or gradual. Patients with fibromyalgia develop tenderness in distinct soft tissue areas—so-called "trigger points" that, when touched, tend to transmit pain to different parts of the body (see diagrams in Chapter 5 for the location of typical trigger points in the different areas of the body). The muscles are taut. The joints, the hands, the feet feel swollen, even though swelling cannot be seen by others.

In fibromyalgia, there is no development of joint destruction, no crippling or deformity. There is, however, significant fatigue, depression, and nervousness. Fibromyalgia may be *primary* (meaning that it can occur alone) or it may be *secondary* to another condition that causes pain or disrupts sleep.

Fibromyalgia causes numbness, tingling, increased pain sensitivity, and a sense of weakness. This sense of weakness is unmeasurable, however, because in objective tests the patient often can exert full force despite the pain. Fibromyalgia can occur with *irritable bowel syndrome, irritable bladder,* and the extreme discomfort that can be associated with menstrual periods. It is also associated with chronic or recurrent migraines and tension headaches.

Of itself, fibromyalgia may last weeks or years, resulting from viral illness, trauma (such as a motor vehicle accident), or excess stress. It may start or remain in a localized pattern—for example, it may limit itself to the neck—or it may spread across the entire body.

Fibromyalgia is closely associated with poor quality, unrefreshing sleep—what is also described as *nonrestorative sleep.* Patients with the condition wake up in the morning more exhausted than when they went to bed. This feeling of extreme fatigue does not ease up in a matter of minutes as normally happens; it may persist for hours. Any poor sleep may precipitate fibromyalgia; on the other hand, the condition itself may lead to poor sleep. Since most patients with fibromyalgia have a poor sleep pattern, it is difficult to know which came first, the fibromyalgia or the sleeping problem. In one sense, it doesn't matter. As the saying goes, "Whether the stone hit the pitcher or the pitcher hit the stone, it's going to be bad for the pitcher." The patient suffering from fibromyalgia often enters a vicious cycle of poor sleep, fatigue, and pain. One interesting research conclusion that bears up the close association between sleep (or lack of it) and fibromyalgia: normal people kept awake for several days develop trigger points similar to those found on patients with fibromyalgia.

Personality also figures in this complicated picture. Fibromyalgia seems to be associated with "perfectionist" personalities. Though this is not always the case, a large percentage of patients with fibromyalgia are individuals highly attuned to detail, who take pride in the ability to perform tasks flawlessly.

Fibromyalgia has existed for many, many years, but it has only been recognized recently. For many, as we found in the case of Michelle, doctor shopping is common. The discomfort, depression, and distress caused by the condition finally win out over the anxiety of perhaps being labelled a hypochondriac.

The proper diagnosis of the disease requires a detailed medical history, a physical examination, and, most importantly, the identification of trigger points. Laboratory evaluations are always completely normal in patients with fibromyalgia unless there is an accompanying disease. Unfortunately, fibromyalgia mimics many muscle, bone, and joint disorders.

While fibromyalgia is very treatable, it is difficult to cure. A large part of the treatment is teaching the patient to recognize that this is a real condition that requires treatment the same way any other medical problem does. Treatment focuses on improving sleep quality, exercising, physical and massage therapy, the use of mild nonnarcotic analgesics, and anti-inflammatory medications. Occasionally psychotherapy is in order as well.

Myositis

Ellen, a 50-year-old homemaker, could not understand the growing weakness she experienced over the past six months. First, she had difficulty standing up from a chair. Now she was having trouble raising her arm to comb her hair. She thought that she was either postmenopausal or simply getting old. In frustration, she sought the aid of her physician.

Fortunately, a blood test revealed an elevation of muscle enzymes. A tiny biopsy specimen of one of her muscles indicated severe inflammation. Treatment with cortisone and later a different immune system suppressant arrested the muscle inflammation and allowed her to function normally once again, though she did lose some measure of her original strength.

Myositis (inflamed muscles) can be caused by a variety of diseases affecting the muscle, bone, and joint. Its effects, regardless of the cause, can be extremely dangerous. As the muscle becomes inflamed, it gradually disintegrates, leaking muscle proteins into the bloodstream. Therefore, it is important to recognize not only the complexity of issues surrounding this condition but the severity of its course, if left untreated.

Polymyositis and Dermatomyositis

Polymyositis means multiple inflamed muscles. *Dermatomyositis* is similar but includes the involvement of the skin. The cause of polymyositis is unclear, although many researchers suggest a viral cause. Others believe that toxoplasma, a protozoan transmitted through cats, is the causative agent of at least some cases of the condition.

Patients with polymyositis develop weakness, fatigue, fever, weight loss, joint pain, and occasionally increased sensitivity to cold, especially of the hands and feet. The fingers may actually turn color, particularly white, blue, and red on exposure to cold. This is called *Raynaud's phenomenon,* though it is not specific to polymyositis and may occur in other connective tissue diseases, including *lupus, rheumatoid arthritis,* and *scleroderma.*

Patients with polymyositis do not necessarily experience pain in the muscles. Weakness, particularly in the muscles of the thighs, neck, and upper arms, is the most common symptom of the disease. Patients often complain of difficulty in getting up from a chair or climbing the stairs. They cannot lift heavy objects and eventually cannot raise their arms or even lift their heads from a pillow. Their voice may become hoarse and they may experience muscle cramping.

The patient may also develop shortness of breath because of weakness in the muscles of the chest wall. Polymyositis may directly affect and destroy lung tissue. The disease may also cause difficulty in swallowing if it affects the muscles of swallowing in the neck and throat, and it can extend into the heart, causing heart muscle weakening and possible heart failure. Polymyositis may also cause abnormal heart rhythms.

Polymyositis affects approximately five people per million each year. The severity of the illness is underscored by the fact that 20 to 30 percent of patients who get the disease will die from it within seven years. The odds are even worse for those in whom the disease affects the heart and lung.

Polymyositis affects two age groups. It affects children age 5 to 15 and adults age 30 to 60. It affects females more frequently than males, and it can develop either abruptly or very gradually.

Dermatomyositis is polymyositis associated with peculiar skin lesions, most notably a purple rash over the top of the finger joints and red patches over the knuckles. Some patients with dermatomyositis develop a red rash and swelling of the eyelids. Dermatomyositis may be associated with the development of a variety of cancers—lung, ovary, breast, intestinal, and leukemia —sometimes within a year of the diagnosis of the dermatomyositis.

Polymyositis and dermatomyositis may be components of another connective tissue disease. When several connective tissue diseases occur together, this is called an *overlap syndrome.* A specific disease called *mixed connective tissue disease* consists of elements *of polymyositis, lupus erythematosus,* and *scleroderma* all in the same unfortunate individual.

The proper diagnosis of polymyositis depends upon the medical history of the individual, the physical exam, and laboratory tests. On physical examination, the muscles of the upper arms, neck, and thighs are weak and occasionally tender when touched. There may be atrophy or wasting in these muscle groups, and the patient may waddle as he or she walks, due to a lack of muscle strength. Blood tests may show an elevation of certain muscle enzymes such as the CPK and aldolase due to muscle destruction and leaching out of these enzymes into the blood. Certain antibody tests may also show positive with this disease. A muscle test called an electromyogram may detect abnormalities in muscle fibers, and muscle biopsies will often show inflammation of the involved muscles.

Treatment of polymyositis consists of the use of medications which suppress the immune system and often include cortisone derivatives. Ninety to 95 percent of patients respond to treatment.

Other Causes of Myositis

Among the many other causes of myositis are *rheumatoid arthritis, scleroderma, lupus, Sjögren's syndrome,* as well as *overlap syndrome* and *mixed connective tissue disease* described above. In addition, certain forms of cancer may produce severe inflammation of the muscles. A condition usually involving the lung called *sarcoidosis* may cause inflammation of the muscles. *Vasculitis* or blood vessel inflammation such as that which occurs with *polyarteritis nodosa* may also cause severe inflammation, while several drugs have been shown to cause myositis. These drugs include lovastatin (and other statin drugs), cimetidine, and penicillamine. Patients diagnosed with myositis should be checked to see if they are taking any of these medications.

Other Causes of Muscle Pain and Weakness

What follows is a summary of many of the numerous causes underlying pain and weakness of the muscles. Further descriptions of many can be found in other sections of this book. Still more detailed information about them can be obtained from your doctor—and should be, if you are concerned.

Various types *of infection* can involve the muscles, including viruses, bacteria, and even parasites. *Trichinosis,* acquired by eating poorly cooked pork, may invade the muscles and cause pain and weakness. Protozoa, such as *toxoplasma,* transmitted via cat excrement, may also invade the muscles.

Tuberculosis has been known to involve the muscles as well. *Lyme disease,* caused by a spirochete transmitted by a tick bite, involves many parts of the body including the muscles.

Numerous *neurologic conditions* may result in pain and/or weakness in the muscles, because the nerves produce the electrical impetus for muscle movement. The spinal cord may be directly involved with *diabetes, polio,* and *amyotrophic lateral sclerosis* (ALS) also known as *Lou Gehrig's disease.* Nerves, pinched by a ruptured disc or by bone at the level of the spinal cord, may produce both pain and weakness in the involved areas. Nerves also can be damaged by various conditions which produce *peripheral neuropathy.* If the damaged nerve is involved with muscle function, there may be weakness and pain. *Parkinson's disease,* a condition involving certain areas of the brain, may result in pain and weakness. Likewise, *multiple sclerosis* and *stroke* may result in weakness and discomfort. Similarly, a poorly understood condition called *reflex sympathetic dystrophy syndrome* (also known as *chronic regional pain syndrome* or *shoulder-hand syndrome)* may produce pain and weakness.

The junction at which a nerve contacts a muscle may be subject to disease. *Myasthenia gravis* is a condition that affects the nerve-muscle junction, causing significant weakness. Two drugs, penicillamine and aminoglycoside antibiotics, may also affect the junction and cause weakness.

Certain forms of cancer, particularly *lymphoma* and *leukemia,* may result in muscle pain or weakness. Tumors, in particular *lung cancer,* may result in a bony condition called *hypertrophic osteoarthropathy,* a condition of very painful bones. This may result in a deep-seated pain that feels as if it were muscular.

The endocrine organs may also produce muscle pain and weakness. A fast *(hyperthyroid)* or a slow *(hypothyroid)* thyroid may produce muscle pain and weakness. Likewise, overactive or underactive parathyroid glands and adrenal glands may also result in muscle pain or weakness. The parathyroid glands produce a hormone to control the body's calcium metabolism. The adrenal gland produces cortisol, the body's natural cortisone. The pituitary gland, which produces growth hormone, may cause enlargement of bone and muscle mass if there is excess production of this hormone. Eventually, these enlarged muscles may become weakened and painful.

Many medications are associated with muscle pain and/or weakness. Muscle may be adversely affected with rifampin, vincristine, cimetidine, chloroquine, clofibrate, colchicine, amphotericin B, tryptophan, cholesterol-lowering drugs (statins) and carbamazepine. The use of cortisone derivatives may cause significant muscle weakness as well. Alcohol has an adverse effect on muscle tissue. Several drugs may cause a drug-induced lupus syndrome that may affect the joints and muscles, causing weakness and pain. These drugs include isoniazid, hydralazine, procainamide, and phenytoin.

Sarcoidosis, an inflammatory condition of unclear cause, usually involves the lung. It may also cause pain or weakness of other muscles as the disease progresses. *Paget's disease* is a condition affecting the bone. Bone remodeling, which takes place throughout the body on a normal and regular basis, is poorly produced in Paget's disease, resulting in weakened and painful bones that are susceptible to breakage. All of the bones are not directly involved; patients often complain of pain and weakness which they attribute to the muscles of the involved limbs.

Connective tissue diseases may be associated with muscle pain or weakness. These diseases include *rheumatoid arthritis, scleroderma, lupus, Sjögren's syndrome* as well as *ankylosing spondylitis. Vasculitis* or inflammatory disease of the blood vessels may be associated with muscle involvement as well.

Certain electrolyte abnormalities may result in weakened or painful muscles. Deficiency of potassium, magnesium, phosphate, and calcium may be detrimental to the muscles. These are further described in chapter 10.

Certain nutritional deficiencies that may result in pain and/ or weakness of muscles, include deficiency of vitamin E and selenium, as well as an excess level of copper in the body. In addition, a generalized weakness has been described with deficiency of vitamin C as well as vitamins Bl, B3, and B6. Generalized weakness may also accompany excess vitamin D. These are further described in chapter 10 in the vitamin and mineral sections.

Certain muscle abnormalities are congenital. The muscles require specialized protein and enzymes to function properly. Several of these enzymes may be lacking or deficient genetically, resulting in pain or weakness whenever the muscle is used. *Muscular dystrophy* is a congenital condition which may result in degeneration of muscle tissue. What is not clearly understood about this disease is how certain forms of muscular dystrophy may first show problems in adult life.

The destruction of muscle obviously can result in pain and weakness. Trauma such as an accident in which the muscle is crushed is but one case. Several addictive substances may cause muscle destruction, including alcohol, heroin, amphetamines, cocaine, and phencyclidine ("angel dust").

Our bodies function in a delicate balance. Normally an intricate interplay among the many organ systems—heart, lung, kidney, thyroid and adrenal glands, etc.—figures in our capacity not only of being well but of *feeling* well. Of no less importance is the need to maintain fairly constant blood and tissue levels of electrolytes and vitamins. Any significant aberration in either these levels or in this greater balance will likely result in lethargy—what you might think of as fatigue, of feeling constantly tired, exhausted and rundown.

Although fatigue is a very nonspecific symptom, it generally points to a significant, often correctable, problem. What is surprising is that so many people simply accept being and feeling tired all the time. They rationalize it as an inevitable consequence of the aging process or the effects of working very hard. To be sure, some degree of weariness does occur with the advancing years, just as too many hours behind a desk can leave you feeling exhausted. However, work and the aging process should be seen as the culprit only after all other suspects have been eliminated. What follows is a summary of some of the more common causes of fatigue.

For reasons that are not entirely clear, chronic illness—that is, illness that is not curable—can cause tiredness or lassitude. *Rheumatoid arthritis* and other connective tissue diseases, *polymyalgia rheumatica,* and *temporal arteritis* and many chronic neurological diseases are just a few of the chronic illnesses often accompanied by a sense of exhaustion. Treatment of the disease in question, curiously, often diminishes the patient's weariness to a noticeable degree.

Chronic infections similarly cause fatigue: *Lyme disease* and *tuberculosis* are just two of many infections that can result in a constant sense of being tired.

Medications themselves very often induce a feeling of sluggishness. Nonsteroidal anti-inflammatory drugs, cortisone, and methotrexate, for example, are used to treat arthritic conditions, but among their side-effects is the tendency to leave the patient feeling run down and sleepy. Others, such as beta-blockers used to treat high blood pressure and angina, very often cause fatigue. Similarly, the common gout medication, allopurinol, can exhaust some patients. Nearly any medication may be responsible; the question is what condition is being treated and what drug is being used to treat it. Observation after stopping medications one at a time in tired patients sometimes can reveal tremendous improvement in energy levels.

Not least among the causes of tiredness are possible psychological causes. *Depression,* for example, is an often overlooked cause of fatigue. Arthritis and other chronic illnesses have emotional as well as physical effects, among them depression. Unfortunately, many patients don't recognize—let alone admit to—their melancholia.

The point here is that the fatigue generated by a sense of despair may perpetuate the debilitating, vicious cycle of chronic illness. It is important to recognize that depression and related psychological conditions that are the side effects of chronic physical illness are quite treatable. What is more, any effective treatment program for the physical condition should take account of the patient's emotional condition as well. Current research is delving into certain chemical imbalances that may precipitate and perpetuate depression and related problems.

Patients who have significant lung, heart, or kidney disease often are fatigued. Lung patients may suffer from an excess of carbon dioxide or a paucity of oxygen in the bloodstream. Consequently, much of their energy is spent in what is termed "the work of breathing," leaving little strength for anything else. Patients with heart disease, on the other hand, may suffer insufficient blood flow to such body areas as the brain or the limbs, resulting in chronic weariness. In addition, heart failure may lead to secondary breathing problems, aggravating the feeling of exhaustion. Patients with significant kidney disease may not be eliminating the body's naturally produced toxins, a condition that can cause a great deal of fatigue. One general effect of dialysis, at least partially, is that it can improve the patient's listlessness.

Chronic pain has always been a very significant source of energy loss, in part due to the chronic depression that inevitably develops. Sometimes, the fatigue is the result of the body and brain efforts to marshal all forces to deal with significant pain constantly. We are only now just beginning to understand what really occurs on a biochemical basis in patients who experience pain every minute of the day.

Certain vitamins and mineral deficiencies have been held to be a source of fatigue. *Vitamin B12* and *folic acid deficiencies* are two conditions believed to cause energy loss, even before each deficiency causes a significant drop in the red blood count *(anemia)*. Vitamin B12 deficiency is quite common—this in spite of the fact that the average diet has sufficient vitamin Bl2. The reason for this is that vitamin B12 absorption in the gut depends upon the production of intrinsic factor from our stomach lining, or parietal cells. The parietal cells may not be producing sufficient intrinsic factor, perhaps because the body has begun to produce antibodies directed against the parietal cells. Another possible cause is the development of antibodies directed against the intrinsic factor itself. It is well known that patients who have had gastrectomy (stomach removal procedure) are prone to develop vitamin B12 deficiency. Most people with significant vitamin B12 deficiency are not able to absorb enough B12 from food and so require intermittent B12 injections. These injections have proven almost totally effective.

One difficult aspect of the problem is that vitamin B12 levels in the blood are not as clearly indicative of vitamin B12 deficiency as we might expect. In fact, significant B12 deficiency can exist though blood levels may be reading as "low normal." Sometimes a trial of vitamin B12 treatment can be most helpful, even if the Bl2 level in the blood is a low normal. However, if B12 deficiency is allowed to continue, it will eventually lead to anemia and sometimes even severe, irreparable nerve damage. Such anemia, called *pernicious anemia,* is completely rectified with periodic injections of B12. The nerve damage is not so easily corrected.

One interesting line of current research suggests that some cases of dementia in the elderly may be due to undetected vitamin B12 deficiency. It also seems that B12 deficiency may be associated with autoantibodies—antibodies directed against one's own body. There are connections between B12 deficiency and several autoantibody diseases, such as *vitiligo* (a lack of pigment in certain areas of the skin), *diabetes, thyroid disease,* and *adrenal gland disease.*

Another problem that can significantly contribute to fatigue is obvious—lack of good quality sleep. Sleep can be described as being either restorative or nonrestorative. Some people can awake exhausted after ten hours of sleep while others may require only several hours to maintain abundant levels of energy. Any cause of sleep disturbance— waking at night from pain or even getting up frequently to go to the bathroom—may result in a serious disruption of restorative sleep.

Physicians have known for a long time that one of the earliest signs of a hidden tumor may be fatigue or depression. Even before the tumor metastasizes or spreads widely throughout the body, the patient loses a great deal of energy. The reasons are not yet clear. There is some speculation that chemical mediators either from the tumor or from the body's response to the tumor produce lethargy in the patient even before the more direct effects of the tumor are experienced. Fatigue may precede the loss of appetite or weight loss which often accompanies many types of tumors. It is important to recognize that the tumor may be in a very localized and curable stage when the patient initially senses the loss of energy.

Numerous electrolyte abnormalities have been cited as causes of fatigue, including abnormalities in sodium, potassium, calcium, magnesium, and phosphate. Correction of the abnormality often improves energy levels significantly. However, it is important to understand the *cause* of the electrolyte abnormality.

Vitamin deficits, in addition to the aforementioned vitamin B12 and folic acid deficiencies, may produce weariness. Lack of vitamin A and vitamin C, for example, has been described as causing fatigue. Several authorities also cite deficiencies in vitamins Bl, B3, and B6 as potential causes of listlessness. Checking vitamin levels in a patient who may be prone to certain types of deficiency may be invaluable.

Endocrine diseases have been recognized for years as being extremely tiring. Classically, *hypothyroidism* or a low thyroid results in significant lethargy. The thyroid gland produces thyroid hormone which regulates the metabolism to a great degree. A low thyroid state is becoming increasingly recognized as a relatively common complaint and should be considered in cases where patients complain of fatigue.

The *adrenal gland* produces the body's own cortisone, called cortisol. Another part of the adrenal gland produces adrenaline. Destruction of adrenal gland tissue can occur with certain diseases, such as tuberculosis, and lead to utter exhaustion. Alternatively, the adrenal gland may be ravaged by the body's own antibodies. Adrenal gland testing may demonstrate that the adrenal glands are producing insufficient hormone. Patients may feel quite weak and have low blood pressure if adrenal gland function is low.

Another endocrine gland which deserves greater attention is the parathyroid gland. There are normally four parathyroid glands in the neck, close to the thyroid gland. The parathryroid gland is responsible for producing parathormone, which in turn is responsible in a large measure for our calcium metabolism. Parathyroid hormone excess or deficiency may result in abnormal calcium levels which may, in turn, affect energy levels. Of the electrolytes, magnesium is particularly responsible for assisting the parathyroid gland to maintain proper blood levels of parathyroid hormone. Consequently, deficiencies of magnesium may lead to abnormalities in the calcium level.

Anemia, which is low blood cell count, can cause significant fatigue by virtue of the function of red blood cells. Red blood cells contain hemoglobin that combines with oxygen absorbed from the lung. This way, oxygen is transported to all tissues of the body. If the blood count is low, less oxygen is being delivered to all body tissue, including the muscles and the brain—hence the fatigue.

Any cause of anemia and any type of anemia will have this effect. This includes iron deficiency anemia, vitamin B12 or folic acid deficiency anemia, and anemia caused by red cell destruction in certain diseases such as *lupus erythematosus.* Other causes of anemia include gastrointestinal bleeding and many arthritic conditions often associated with the chronic disease anemia. Some useful medications are available to improve anemia in the presence of kidney and other chronic diseases. A synthetic protein called erythropoietin is produced by advanced gene cloning techniques in bacteria, resulting in the ability to make the substance in sufficient quantities for use in humans. This protein has potential for improving anemia; therefore, it should also have an effect on the energy levels of patients suffering from more severe chronic anemias.

Frequently overlooked as a cause of lassitude is the lack of regular exercise. Lifestyle change, time constraints, inability to exercise due to muscle or joint pain all may lead to a sedentary existence. Simply working, even in a physically demanding job, won't adequately tax the heart, muscles, and joints to be of sufficient benefit. The payoff of even a mild but regular exercise regime is enormous, resulting in a dramatic increase in energy levels.

Another cause of fatigue, perhaps as obvious as the loss of restorative sleep, is significant weight gain. Weight gain can, of course, be associated with a number of different conditions, including *depression, low thyroid state,* and increased energy requirements in general. Part of the weight problem has to do with social demands and expectations. We place such emphasis on the pleasurable aspects of eating that eating itself for many people—regardless of *what* they're eating—becomes a reward. Overindulgence is gratifying, socially acceptable, and an easy trap when a person does not have mastery over other delights in life.

On the other side of things, we tend to be rather unforgiving in our treatment of people with weight problems. Often, the admonition for being overweight becomes a reason for eating more. And in many cases when people with weight problems attempt to diet, they experience wide vacillations of weight gain and weight loss. Recent findings indicate the danger of dramatic variations of weight in the individual, particularly in terms of heart disease. That having been said, losing weight will improve energy levels by "easing the load" an individual must carry. Among the factors that perpetuate overindulgence leading to fatigue are depression and any physical condition that inhibits physical activity.

Side effects of certain medications can sometimes lead to significant weight gain. Some medications used to treat arthritic conditions, for example, may increase appetite. Other medications may provoke a "sweet tooth," and still others leave such a dreadful aftertaste that a patient will do anything to block it. A low thyroid state as described above may reduce energy supplies and in addition may lead to excessive weight gain.

Any weight loss program, to be effective in the long term, must address directly those factors contributing to overindulgence and the difficulties individuals sometimes face in finding alternative forms of enjoyment and gratification. Conditions which adversely affect caloric expenditure must be examined and dealt with when possible. Generally, weight loss and weight gain is part of a larger picture— what is all too often a vicious cycle. For example, chronic arthritic conditions may lead to physical inactivity; chronic pain in turn promotes loss of self-esteem and depression. Lack of ability to function physically and perhaps sexually leads to closing of important outlets for gratification. Total body weight increases due to the inability to expend calories, which propagates further depression and lethargy which, in turn, leads to continued overindulgence.

Delineating the cause of fatigue is complicated—sometimes painful, sometimes difficult to track simply because of the complexity of systemic problems. The compensation, however, is *always* worth it. Even multiple causes are for the greater part highly treatable. Careful attention to detail and the consultation of a concerned health care professional will help greatly in defining the origins of a patient's fatigue.

Now that you have had the chance to see not only what arthritis *is* but also what arthritis *isn't,* let's look at some related diseases. Primary among these are the CORE diseases—those ailments akin to arthritis that affect the bones, muscles, and joints. The CORE diseases (Crystal diseases, Osteoarthritis, Rheumatoid diseases, Enthesopathies) are those that often cause musculoskeletal pain. See Table 1.

Table 1 – CORE diseases	
Crystal diseases	Gout
	Pseudogout
	other calcium deposition diseases
Osteoarthritis	also known as degenerative joint disease
Rheumatoid arthritis and other connective tissue diseases	
	Sjögren's syndrome
	Lupus erythematosus
	Scleroderma
	Polymyositis & dermatomyositis
	Mixed connective tissue disease
	Overlap syndromes
Enthesopathies	Ankylosing spondylitis
	Psoriatic arthritis
	Reactive arthritis
	Inflammatory bowel arthritis

Crystal diseases are those, like gout, that leave crystal deposits in the spaces within and surrounding the joints. These crystal deposits cause the extraordinary pain associated with crystal diseases.

Osteoarthritis is generally held to be "old age wear and tear." It is a degenerative joint disease that most often appears in individuals over the age of 50.

Rheumatoid diseases are autoimmune—that is, they originate in the body's mechanism for fighting infection and other foreign entities. The effect of these diseases is generally widespread throughout the body, causing inflammation in the kidney, the joints, the skin, and even in the brain on occasion. Along with *rheumatoid arthritis,* this category includes *lupus, scleroderma,* and *polymyositis.*

Enthesopathies are those diseases that affect the tendons and ligaments, particularly where they attach to the bone. Enthesopathies apparently are of genetic origin—90% of patients with *ankylosing spondylitis,* for example, have a genetic marker called HLA B27. The diseases are characterized by an inflammation of ligaments, tendons, and joints.

Crystal Diseases

Gout

Gout is different from other types of arthritis because it involves the deposition of uric acid crystals (hence its inclusion among the crystal diseases) in and around the joint space. While the disease was commonly diagnosed and depicted as far back as the 17th century, one sure way to make its diagnosis is to find uric acid crystals in the joint fluid. Alternatively, a newer technology, musculoskeletal ultrasound, may show a picture that is very distinct for gout.

The pain in gout is actually produced by the white blood cells in the body and not the uric acid crystals directly. White blood cells are designed to fight foreign material, and while they correctly detect the deposits in the joint, it is actually their presence, as attackers of the uric acid crystals, that causes the severe pain, tenderness, redness, and swelling found in an acute attack of gout.

129

Anyone who has experienced such an attack will tell you it is one of the most painful things they have ever endured. The depiction of the gout victim in 17th and 18th century art suggests the disfavor with which the disease has been regarded, which continues today. The subject is always a wealthy, corpulent man sitting at a table heavily laden with rich foods and drink. His big toe is wrapped up in a silk bandage and elevated prominently on some plump cushions. The image, and it is one that taints victims of gout to this very day, is one of gross consumption.

But while diet and excessive drinking can aggravate gout in an individual, the person must already have a tendency toward the disease. In any case, diet is not its primary cause. As noted before, gout can be diagnosed absolutely when uric acid crystals have been observed in the joint fluid. A drop of fluid is removed from an involved joint and is immediately examined under a special polarizing microscope set for specific visualization of the uric acid crystals.

Many times, the physician must make the diagnosis based on other factors of the disease. For example, most patients with gout have high levels of uric acid in their blood. Unfortunately, excess uric acid in the blood can signify many different things. The kidney may not be removing the uric acid efficiently from the bloodstream, for instance, or the patient may have a genetic disorder which inclines him (or her, though as a recessive trait, it is most often found among men) toward excessive production of uric acid in the metabolism. For others, excess uric acid is a side-effect of medications, such as diuretics or "water pills" which are often used to lower blood pressure or eliminate excess body fluids. These and other medications cause *hyperuricemia* (elevated uric acid level in the blood) either by interfering with the excretion of uric acid or by provoking its overproduction in the body.

Finally, excess uric acid may be associated with other diseases which involve a rapid turnover of cells—*leukemia* (a cancer of white blood cells), for example, or *psoriasis* (a skin disease). Increased cell reproduction results in a marked increase in the production of purines, later metabolized to uric acid.

But before we chastise the artist who painted the overindulgent gentleman for not being true to life, excess uric acid production is seen in the obese as well as the alcoholic. That having been said, a high uric acid level in the blood does not mean that the patient *will* have gout; nor will all patients with gout necessarily have high uric acid levels in their blood. The question remains whether there are uric acid crystals present in the joint fluid.

Another suggestion of gout is the presence of tophi, soft collections of uric acid crystals and debris in the tissue. Frequently, this occurs at the edge of the ear, at the elbows, or over the joints. These soft tissue nodules can be distinguished from others which occur with different types of arthritis (like the rheumatoid nodules that can be found in rheumatoid arthritis) because they contain uric acid and the others do not. Gouty nodules may cause severe joint damage and erosion when they are present over a joint. They may also break and ooze uric acid and debris. When the overlying skin is broken, they may become infected.

Over one million people in the United States have gout. Between seventy and ninety percent of those affected are middle-aged men. Most victims of the disease have several attacks, though a single attack in a lifetime is possible. The most common kind of gout attack involves the big toe, bringing on a symptom known as *podagra,* where the toe becomes very suddenly and very extremely painful and red. The pain is, in the technical sense of the term, *exquisite*—that is, so bad that even the weight of a bedsheet can cause excruciating suffering. Typically, an attack will involve only one joint, generally in the lower extremities—the big toe, the ankle, the knee. Gout may also involve tendons and soft tissues, such as the top or side of the foot. The attack starts quickly and peaks very rapidly.

For unclear reasons, gout rarely involves the shoulders, although it may eventually involve the elbow, wrist, and hand joints. It is important to remember that if a patient suffers a number of gout attacks, they will not necessarily involve the same joint, nor will they necessarily be restricted to a single joint at any one time. Gout has been known to strike upper and lower extremities simultaneously.

Lastly, gout can occur in any situation that causes a rapid change in uric acid levels. For example, diarrhea and other types of dehydration can lead to an attack. Even certain medications used to *lower* uric acid may precipitate a gouty attack if the uric acid level is lowered rapidly. Similarly, surgery and severe medical illness have been known to induce an attack.

Can gout be cured? As advances are made in the treatment of the genetic disposition, this disease, which seems to be related primarily to a defect in the metabolism of purines to uric acid, will ultimately be controlled fully. In the meantime, conventional medicine does provide adequate means for the treatment of the symptoms.

Pseudogout (CPPD Disease)

Another type of crystal-induced arthritis was only recognized in the early '60s. Often referred to as *pseudogout* or *calcium pyrophosphate dihydrate crystal deposition disease* (CPPD disease, for short), this disease can take many forms. Crystals may precipitate in the joint fluid as in gout, or be deposited in the cartilage of the joints themselves, causing a condition known as *chondrocalcinosis.*

These calcifications can occur in the hyaline cartilage, the cartilage of the joint surface itself. Crystal deposition may also take place in the cartilage of tendon and the ligamentous attachments to the bone (the entheses).

Most patients with CPPD disease also have other types of arthritis. The deposition of CPPD crystals may occur in a joint already damaged by osteoarthritis, rheumatoid arthritis, or any other form of arthropathy. Indeed, when CPPD disease occurs in combination with other arthritic conditions, it is sometimes difficult to determine how much disability and joint pain is due to each component. CPPD disease also is often associated with several metabolic and endocrine abnormalities, such as excess iron deposition *(hemochromatosis)* and magnesium deficiencies. *Diabetes mellitus,* a disease that interferes with the regulation of glucose (sugar) metabolism, can occur with CPPD disease.

Unfortunately, the list of associations with CPPD disease does not end there. It can occur with *hypothyroidism* (underactive thyroid function) and *hyperparathyroidism* (abnormal calcium metabolism).

Whatever its associations, CPPD disease is definitely not related to a dietary overabundance of calcium. Rather, it may stem from an over accumulation of pyrophosphate, a normal byproduct of tissue destruction. The discovery of a rare congenital form of CPPD disease lends support to this theory.

CPPD disease, given its nickname *pseudogout* (false gout), shares certain traits with gout itself. Most notably, its diagnosis is demonstrated by the presence of crystals in the joint fluid. CPPD occurs most commonly in the knee, wrist, hip and shoulder. It may also affect the elbow, ankle, and small joints of the hand. In the last case, it may imitate *rheumatoid arthritis* (a condition then justly called *pseudo rheumatoid arthritis*). CPPD disease differs from gout in that it affects men and women equally, especially the elderly. Frequently, it occurs in the sixth or seventh decade and affects roughly five percent of the adult population. However, it is present, according to pathologic surveys, in 50 percent of the population over age 90.

This disease may occur in an acute form very similar to gout, with its characteristically sudden onset of pain, redness, and swelling. It can last from several days to several weeks and disappear, even without specific treatment. In chronic form, it can affect several joints at once and persist for longer periods of time. The joint changes often progress rapidly and are very severe. In some ways, CPPD disease is similar to osteoarthritis (see below), but there is more destructive change and cyst formation. Physical activity often makes the problem much worse.

Treatment depends on the severity of symptoms. Joint aspiration to remove crystals often gives some relief, and the injection of corticosteroids directly into the joint can relieve the problem. Nonsteroidal anti-inflammatory agents, however, are the mainstay of treatment, though colchicine has been used to some effect. Rest, the protection of affected joints with splints, and the use of ambulatory aides is recommended during periods of active disease. Exercise is recommended after the flare subsides to maintain range of motion and build strength.

Osteoarthritis (Degenerative Joint Disease)

This type of arthritis is probably present in varying degrees in all adults over the age of 60. According to X-ray surveys, at least ten percent of all adults have moderate or severe joint degeneration attributable to this disease, although the degree of change indicated on X-rays does not always correlate with the amount of pain or disability. Approximately seventy-five percent of patients classified as severely disabled by arthritis have primarily *osteoarthritis*. Unlike many other forms of arthritis, osteoarthritis affects only the joints and manifests itself in symptoms affecting the joint, the cartilage, the underlying bones, and the related muscles. Patients with osteoarthritis may experience joint pain, tenderness, stiffness, and limited motion. There may be an accumulation of fluid in the joint space; patients may also feel or hear crepitus or "creaking" in the joint. The muscles surrounding the affected joints may become atrophied or wasted from disuse over an extended period of time.

Osteoarthritis has no general systemic effects associated with it, such as fever, chills, weight loss, or anemia. The onset of symptoms is gradual, involving progressive loss of function. Pain tends to be aggravated by use of the involved joint and ameliorated with rest. The patient may feel morning stiffness, but this lasts only briefly, perhaps ten minutes or so. Stiffness tends to recur after any period of inactivity.

Those most likely to be affected by osteoarthritis are persons aged over

50. When the disease strikes before age 50, victims are more often men than women, because, it is speculated, men are exposed to more joint trauma in their work and in their leisure activities. Over age 55, however, the reverse is true: osteoarthritis affects women three times as often as it affects men. One form of the disease, called *erosive* or *inflammatory osteoarthritis*, usually occurs in Caucasian women after the onset of menopause, causing severe, erosive, and deforming changes primarily in the hands. Inflammatory osteoarthritis seems to be genetically based.

As for "garden-variety" osteoarthritis, the primary form of the disease may occur in a localized form, affecting the knees or hips, the hands, or the spine. It may also take a generalized form, involving three or more joint groups, including the distal and proximal finger and toe joints, the knees, the shoulders, and the feet. It may also involve the ankle, elbow, and the wrist.

One of the factors that can make osteoarthritis difficult to diagnose is its occurrence in association with other forms of arthritis. For example, a *crystal disease, pseudogout,* commonly occurs in joints already damaged by osteoarthritis. Similarly, major joint injury to the bone underlying the joint cartilage is felt to predispose to later osteoarthritis. Surgical removal of a damaged meniscus (cartilage cushion of the knee joint) may be followed some 10 to 20 years later by development of osteoarthritis. Congenital abnormalities, such as a dislocated hip or unequal leg length, can also predispose the individual to osteoarthritis. Finally, osteoarthritis has sometimes been associated with certain metabolic and endocrine disorders, such as *hypothyroidism.*

The first changes occurring in the joint affected by osteoarthritis are marked by an irregular loss in the cartilage layer. This appears in X-rays as a narrowing of the joint space, particularly in areas of stress. As the adjacent bone attempts to repair the joint, it first becomes denser or *sclerotic* in the areas of the damaged cartilage. Bony outgrowths called *osteophytes* (spurs) tend to form as a result, distorting the surface of the joint. Cysts may also form in the bone.

With these outgrowths and cysts, the lining of the joint space (the *synovium)* becomes inflamed, further reducing the functional capacity of the joint.

The diagnosis of osteoarthritis is made through the evaluation of the patient's medical history and a complete physical examination. Confirmation comes with X-rays. Laboratory tests generally show no abnormalities, but as noted above, osteoarthritis is often associated with the crystal diseases, so examination of the joint fluid in the affected areas may be warranted.

Treatment is initially geared toward education and pain relief. At first, the patient needs to learn how to help him- or herself. Occupational therapy can provide the means to improve function in daily living, whether it involves the use of button hooks and zipper pulls for grasping and pulling, to learning how to use a walker or crutches. At times, the patient will need outside help with meals and other necessities.

Physical therapy is another element in the treatment plan to improve joint function and diminish pain by maintaining joint mobility and strength as much as possible. In obese patients, a course in weight reduction is strongly advised, as the overweight patient carries an extraordinary and unnecessary load, which often further damages the already injured joints.

At this time, medications are used primarily for pain relief. The basis for most drug treatment is the nonsteroidal anti-inflammatory drugs (NSAID's). These can provide not only pain relief, they can also act on the inflammation in the osteoarthritic joint. Acetaminophen, though widely used, has minimal efficacy as a treatment for osteoarthritis. It must be mentioned that nonsteroidal anti-inflammatory drugs have a host of potential toxicities that limit their use. These include potential damage to the liver, kidneys, and lining of the stomach leading to bleeding. Most important, there is an increased risk of cardiovascular events such as heart attack and stroke.

The patient may require stronger pain relief medication. Steroid injections may be used for local relief in a particularly affected joint. Frequent injections – more often than three times per year are not indicated, however, as they may actually contribute to further joint destruction. Viscosupplement injections are lubricants that may be beneficial for symptomatic relief of osteoarthritis of the knee. All injections should be administered using ultrasound guidance to ensure accuracy.

Surgical options, from arthroscopic surgery to joint replacement, are considered only when the patient is continually suffering severe pain, restriction of movement, or has an unstable joint. Several new treatments are currently being developed to treat the cartilage itself by preventing further destruction of the tissue and, perhaps, even allowing for the possibility of repair. Examples include cartilage growth factors such as mesenchymal stem cells.

Rheumatoid Diseases

Rheumatoid diseases are superficially diverse, but they all are *autoimmune diseases*. In other words, they are the products of the very defense mechanism the body has to protect itself from infection and other foreign invaders.

Normally, when the body identifies a foreign presence, it produces and sends antibodies and other proteins to destroy, for example, the infection, tumor, or cancer. Together, these antibodies and proteins are called immune complexes. However, something happens—we are not yet quite sure—that turns these antibodies against the body itself. The result is that deposits of these immune complexes can appear in such different places as the filtration system of the kidney, the joints, the skin, and even, in some circumstances, the brain. The action of these complexes effectively inflames the affected area, bringing about the symptoms we identify as the *rheumatoid diseases*.

Perhaps the best known of these is ***rheumatoid arthritis.*** Generally thought of as "bad kind of arthritis," the truth is that like all the diseases in this category, *rheumatoid arthritis* can be very debilitating, but it is often found in mild forms. It is a systemic disease; that is, it affects the entire body as well as the joints. It is also relatively common, affecting about one percent of the population.

As with most autoimmune diseases, rheumatoid arthritis usually begins between the ages of 20 and 50. Only ten to fifteen percent of patients are over age 50 at the onset of the disease; another five percent of patients are children under the age of 16. Women are affected about three times as often as men.

Recent research indicates a genetic predisposition to this form of arthritis and the related autoimmune diseases. In rheumatoid arthritis, an antigen called HLA DR4 occurs on the surface of the white blood cells more frequently in affected patients, occurring in seventy percent of white patients with the disease but in less than thirty percent of white patients without it. Among African Americans there is a similar spread, with HLA DR4 occurring in almost fifty percent of those suffering from rheumatoid arthritis and in less than fifteen percent of those without it.

The role of this genetic product is not certain, especially since the presence or absence of HLA DR4 antigen is not by itself proof of the disease. Current thinking is that this genetic product may alter the immune response. According to this theory, rheumatoid arthritis is the result of an abnormal response to the action of an unknown infectious agent instead of, or in addition to, an immune response against the self.

About 70 percent of rheumatoid arthritis patients produce a specific antibody called *rheumatoid factor.* This is, in effect, an antibody that attacks other antibodies. Rheumatoid factor therefore is an "autoantibody." Interestingly, as people age, they normally produce more autoantibodies, including rheumatoid factor. Increasing numbers of autoantibodies are also produced with chronic infections. Thus, it is very common to find a very small amount or "titer" of rheumatoid factor present in patients who do not have rheumatoid arthritis; higher amounts are usually, though not always, associated with active rheumatoid arthritis. A more specific antibody found in patients with RA is the anti-CCP. A patient with the combination of a positive rheumatoid factor and a positive anti-CCP almost assuredly has rheumatoid arthritis.

Other autoantibodies are sometimes seen in rheumatoid arthritis, notably *antinuclear antibody* (ANA). This is especially the case in the juvenile form of rheumatoid arthritis. Most patients with rheumatoid arthritis have a generalized increase in their levels of many other antibodies, as though their immune systems had been awakened without much sense of what specifically had disturbed them.

While the theory behind the development of rheumatoid arthritis is still very much in its early stages, the effects of the disease in the joint have been extensively studied. Immune complexes appear in the lining of the joint. The lining cells of the joint space (the *synovium)* become swollen and inflamed, extending into and around the joint space itself. This overgrowth of tissue can cause a boggy or doughy consistency to the joint.

As the inflamed synovium extends, it erodes the articular cartilage and tendons, causing further disruption of the joint and the destructive deformity so often associated with rheumatoid arthritis. A secondary inflammatory response then causes further swelling, redness, heat, and pain. Usually, joint manifestations of rheumatoid arthritis start in the peripheral joints and tendon sheaths. In the more common polyarticular (multiple-joint) form of the disease, the small joints of the hands and feet are involved symmetrically—both the left and the right wrists, for example. In the hands, the disease generally attacks the knuckles more frequently than the distal portion of the fingers. It eventually spreads to larger joints, such as the knee, but may involve other joints, including the ankle, wrist, elbow, shoulder, and hip.

Rheumatoid arthritis is more than just a joint disease. It is a multisystem disorder and can attack internal organs. About thirty percent of patients with the disease develop lumps called *rheumatoid nodules* which are masses of inflammatory cells. These nodules are often seen at the elbow and can be particularly irritating when present on the palm of the hand. They also may be present in the internal organs, such as the heart and the lungs.

Rheumatoid arthritis also brings with it a number of nonspecific, systemic problems. Patients often experience weight loss, fatigue, fever, muscle wasting, and anemia. Patients may say that they feel "just plain rotten." They may also suffer an inflammation of the *pleura* (sac covering the lungs) or of the *pericardium* (sac covering the heart). Burning, tingling, or numbness of the hands and feet *(peripheral neuropathy)* is common; the eyes often suffer dryness and *keratoconjunctivitis,* an irritation of the superficial layer of the eye tissue. *Scleritis,* the irritation of the white of the eye, may also occur.

A dangerous possible manifestation of rheumatoid arthritis is *vasculitis,* an inflammation of the blood vessels. This appears as painful redness, with sores at the fingertips and the toes and can develop to gangrene if left untreated. Another potential hazard with rheumatoid arthritis is *Felty's syndrome,* which combines rheumatoid arthritis with an enlarged spleen. In this case, the patient has a very low white blood count, which renders him or her particularly susceptible to infection.

As if these problems weren't enough, other conditions beyond the scope of this book may accompany rheumatoid arthritis. And rheumatoid arthritis is not just for adults; children may suffer its ravages as well. With such a long and varied list of characteristics and possible associated problems, how is it possible to make a definitive diagnosis of rheumatoid arthritis? In 2010 the American College of Rheumatology (ACR) and the European League Against Rheumatism (EULAR) proposed a set of criteria for identifying the disease. These criteria will detect more than 80% of patient with rheumatoid arthritis if a patient certain criteria based upon the history, physical examination and laboratory tests. A definitive diagnosis is still not as easy to make as we would like. Future classification and diagnostic criteria may incorporate musculoskeletal ultrasound as well as magnetic resonance imaging (MRI) which should help improve accuracy.

Treatment of rheumatoid arthritis is directed toward control of pain and inflammation; however, maintaining and restoring function in the joints are also crucial treatment goals. Patients often require the same social adaptation and adjustment that go with other chronic and disabling diseases.

Anti-inflammatory medications including salicylates and nonsteroidal anti-inflammatory drugs (NSAIDs) are the first level of treatment. Many patients will respond better to one or the other, and if there is no relief of symptoms at an adequate dose, medications will likely be switched. Steroids (cortisone) taken by mouth almost always gain control of the disease, but the side effects of large doses over long periods of time can be quite serious. Even in low doses, steroids may predispose the patient to *osteoporosis,* infection, and other complications. Steroid injections straight into the joint may be effective, but only if the flare involves a single joint.

Other possible treatments involve the use of remittive or disease-modifying antirheumatic drugs (DMARDs). One of the most effective DMARDS for treatment of rheumatoid arthritis is methotrexate. This is the "workhorse" and is probably the most widely used DMARD. Other lesser known DMARDS include hydroxychloroquine (Plaquenil®), leflunomide (Arava®), and sulfasalazine (Azulfidine®).

While some rheumatologists advocate the use of combination DMARDS to treat rheumatoid arthritis, we have not found it to be that effective.

Biologic agents, first introduced in the late 1990s, have become an important mainstay of treatment of rheumatoid arthritis. These drugs are designed to target the specific abnormalities of the immune system seen in rheumatoid arthritis. Adequate monitoring

141

of all these agents, however, is essential. The above agents may be used alone (monotherapy) or in combination. The goal is to improve inflammation, pain, and function but also to slow or stop joint destruction and even prolong life since rheumatoid arthritis and many other inflammatory conditions increase the proclivity toward premature cardiovascular disease. Effective treatment may decrease the risk of premature death from stroke and heart attack.

Physical therapy is a crucial part of the treatment plan. Local modalities, such as heat and ice, may help control pain and inflammation. Splints are often needed to rest an acutely inflamed joint and to help avoid deformity. Range of motion exercises in all joints, especially those acutely involved, help to maintain function.

When deformity and disability have occurred, there are many devices which can enable the patient to care for him- or herself and function independently. These vary from built-up utensils to button hooks and other imaginative devices that easily assist the individual to perform the functions of daily living.

And though the issues of diet in the treatment of rheumatoid arthritis are still being evaluated, the patient should maintain a nutritious diet. Please see chapter 10, "Vitamins, Minerals, Diet, and Nutrition."

Finally, family and social support are crucial in the management of this chronic disease. One of the physician's key roles is often to help the patient's family adjust to the sometimes dramatic changes in the individual's functional abilities. Education of the patient, the family, and the community will allow the patient to achieve his or her fullest potential.

Systemic lupus erythematosus (SLE or just *lupus)* is another autoimmune disease. In this disease, protein antibodies attack such self-components as evidenced by the production of antinuclear antibodies and antiDNA antibodies. The difficulty with this disease is its dramatically different manifestations from patient to patient. One patient may have only mild skin involvement, some joint pain, and abnormal lab tests, while another may have convulsions, kidney failure, or a loss of touch with reality.

How can a disease with such diverse manifestations be diagnosed? Rheumatologists have been trying to decide how to define or *classify* the disease statistically, based on a set of criteria. These are for including or excluding patients for studies and not strictly for diagnostic purposes.

The *diagnosis* of lupus should be made based upon an evaluation and opinion by an expert rheumatologist.

There are various *classification criteria* which include the following information:

1. *Malar rash*—a butterfly-shaped rash across the bridge of the nose and cheeks.
2. *Discoid rash*—red raised patches with scaling and scarring.
3. *Photosensitivity*—rashes or unusual reactions to sunlight.
4. *Oral (mouth)* or *nasal (nose) ulcers*—shallow sores in the mouth.
5. *Alopecia* (hair loss) without scar formation
6. *Arthritis*—joint pain and swelling, usually involving two or more joints.
7. *Serositis*—inflammation of the sacs surrounding either the heart or the lungs. Pleurisy and pericarditis fall into this category.
8. *Renal (kidney) disorder*—protein or cellular casts in the urine due to kidney dysfunction.
9. *Neurological disorder*—seizures (convulsions) or psychosis.
10. *Hematologic (blood) disorder*—low white blood cell count, low platelet count, or low red blood count (due to red cell destruction).
11. *Immunologic disorder*—specific antibodies in the blood

including antiDNA antibody, antiSm antibody, lupus anticoagulant test, anticardiolipin antibodies, direct Coombs test, low complement, or a false positive test for syphilis.

12. *Antinuclear antibody ("ANA") in the blood*—in the absence of drugs known to cause drug-induced lupus syndrome.

The prevalence of SLE is climbing, possibly because physicians are becoming increasingly aware of its variable manifestations and course. The diagnosis, as a result, is being considered more often and more appropriately. Estimates of its frequency run between 20 and 150 per 100,000, and SLE affects ten times as many women as men. The disease is most common during the childbearing years, but it can occur at any time.

Hormones seem to play an important role in the disease. Flares may occur around the time of pregnancy; they can also be precipitated by the administration of hormones. Young women already diagnosed with the disease are advised to avoid birth control pills. SLE also seems to be more common among particular racial groups, especially African Americans. It clearly shows a higher incidence in certain families, but inheritance is not completely predictable. Not all children or grandchildren will be affected in a family at risk, but more children in such a family will be found to have SLE or a related disease than in other families.

Certain environmental factors may trigger either the disease or a flare, most notably sunlight. Some drugs have been shown to produce a lupus-like syndrome or precipitate a disease flare in patients with known SLE

One factor that may shed important light on the nature of the disease is the fact that an increase in the characteristic autoantibodies has been found in the married partners of patients with SLE as well as in laboratory workers who handle blood specimens from lupus patients. Such findings raise the question as to whether there are viral or other infectious triggers to this disease that we have yet to discover.

Given this extraordinary set of variables, it can hardly be surprising that the progression of SLE is very complicated. The disease may naturally wax and wane, though with appropriate treatment, the disease may go into complete remission for an extended length of time. Unfortunately, this is not always the case. Successful management of SLE requires careful monitoring. An active patient should be seen fairly frequently, with a close follow-up of blood urine tests as well as clinical evaluation. An inactive patient should be followed less frequently to assess disease activity and, hopefully, to avoid the surprise of an unsuspected flare. Patients are counselled to avoid intense sun exposure, wear appropriate clothing, and use high-factor sun screens. SLE patients are taught to get plenty of rest and not to overextend themselves during the day. Infections of any kind are taken very seriously, especially when the patient is undergoing immunosuppressive therapy. Up-to-date immunizations are suggested. Use of hormones (as in birth control pills) can be used if needed if the disease is stable but is an important decision that needs to be made on an individual basis. Any change in the physical condition should be reported immediately to the physician.

Education is crucial with SLE, as it is a potentially lifelong problem. The patient must learn to communicate with both physician and caregivers. Support groups are often helpful to patients with this type of chronic problem, because they can increase the individual's awareness of the disease and the ways in which people learn to manage it.

Scleroderma or *progressive systemic sclerosis* is another autoimmune-based disease, affecting not only skin and joints but the entire system. Since this disease shares many characteristics with SLE, *polymyositis-dermatomyositis,* and *mixed connective tissue disease,* proper diagnosis is sometimes difficult. As with the other connective tissue diseases, the exact cause of scleroderma is unknown. However, certain environmental and physical factors are occasionally implicated as causing scleroderma or a scleroderma-like illness. These include gadolinium-based MRI contrast agents, rapeseed oil, L-tryptophan, and the chemical polyvinyl chloride.

Generally central to the diagnosis of *progressive systemic sclerosis* is skin thickening, though there is a form of the disease in which the skin involvement is minimal. Secondary criteria for the diagnosis of the disease include *sclerodactyly* (fingers with thickened and bound-down skin) loss of fingertip pad tissue, and an abnormal chest X-ray showing lung disease. Patients often exhibit *Raynaud's phenomenon,* in which fingers and toes turn blue when exposed to the cold.

In a limited form of systemic sclerosis called *CREST syndrome,* patients all have Raynaud's phenomenon and sclerodactyly as well as *telangiectasias,* in which fine vessels enlarge and appear like spiderwebs in the skin. In another limited form of this disease, the involvement may be restricted to the skin.

Approximately 250 per million persons experience some form of systemic sclerosis, so it is quite uncommon. The disease is all the more rare in children, reaching its peak onset between ages 45 and 64- There is a two- to three-fold increase of the disease in women.

While the early stages of the disease are nonspecific, the characteristic tightening of the skin on the face and mouth, which makes it difficult for the patient to open the mouth or even smile, may be the first sign. With the accompanying Raynaud's phenomenon and the enlargement of the fine vessels in the skin, the current thinking about systemic sclerosis is that the disease causes a change in the tiny blood vessels. Almost all patients with scleroderma are found to have antinuclear antibodies; anticentromere antibodies are associated with the limited forms of the disease.

Scleroderma often involves the lungs, usually with a condition called *diffuse interstitial fibrosis,* scarring of the lung tissue. Patients frequently complain of shortness of breath and dry cough. Involvement of other internal organs can cause serious complications. Kidney involvement often leads to high blood pressure and in the past has been almost uniformly fatal. Heart complications range from inflammation of the lining of the heart to scarring and thickening of the heart itself, causing abnormal conduction of electrical impulses which in turn leads to sometimes fatal abnormal heart rhythms. Decreased motility of the esophagus (the tube from the mouth to the stomach) and the entire bowel leads to difficulty in swallowing and defecating. Muscle inflammation as well as burning, tingling, and numbness of the hands and feet may occur.

Treatment of this disease in the main focuses on the symptoms. Lung involvement, for example, is often treated with oxygen when necessary. At the present time, severe lung scarring is not reversible, though the kidney complications have been treated by a variety of agents with good success.

Polymyositis and *dermatomyositis* are inflammatory disorders of the muscle. Inflammation of the muscle tissue or *myositis* leads first to weakness. Usually all muscle groups are affected, but involvement of the muscles of the thighs and upper arms occurs first, with patients complaining of the inability to climb stairs, rise from a chair, or even lift an object. They may also experience difficulty in swallowing, speech, and breathing. The disease is often accompanied by a rash over the eyes, neck, chest, and the tops of the hands. This is another rare disease, occurring with roughly five new cases per million population yearly. The problem is most common in African American women. More information can be found in chapter 6, *Muscle pain and weakness.*

Sjögren's syndrome is another autoimmune disease. This causes *dry eyes* and dry *mouth. Dry mouth* is called *xerostomia.* This condition can cause severe difficulties in chewing and swallowing and even in speech. Sores occur in the mouth, and dental cavities are common. This condition is seen in normal aging to a limited degree, but together with *dry eyes (xerophthalmia)* makes up the *sicca syndrome.* The *dry eyes* develop when the lacrimal (tear) glands are destroyed by a connective tissue disease. Damage to the cornea and blindness may occur.

The *sicca syndrome,* that is, *dry eyes* and *dry mouth,* is commonly found

147

in *rheumatoid arthritis, lupus,* and *scleroderma. Sicca syndrome,* however, is primarily thought of in association with *Sjögren's syndrome.*

In *Sjögren's syndrome,* there is salivary gland inflammation and often enlargement. There may be involvement of the muscle, nerve, liver, lung, and kidney. There is an increased association *of Sjögren's syndrome* with *lymphoma,* a kind of malignancy. Enlarged lymph nodes may also occur with *pseudolymphoma,* a benign condition. *Sjögren's syndrome* may occur alone or in association with other connective tissue disorders, including *rheumatoid arthritis, lupus, scleroderma, polymyositis,* and *dermatomyositis.*

Enthesopathies

The fourth group of our CORE diseases is the enthesopathies. These diseases have been called *seronegative spondyloarthropathies* and include *ankylosing spondylitis, psoriatic arthritis, enteropathic arthritis,* and *reactive arthritis.* In the past, they were thought to be variants of rheumatoid arthritis, with an absent or "negative" blood (or serum) factor—hence the classification, "seronegative."

The general site of these diseases is the enthesis area where ligaments or tendons attach to bone. The *enthesopathy* develops with inflammation at these points of attachment. These areas attempt to repair themselves with new bone (spur) formation. With continued bone formation, the entire ligament can become replaced by bone. When this happens in the back or neck, the bones can become fused or *ankylosed.*

Enthesopathies appear to be more common in some families and ethnic groups. There is a genetic marker found on the surface of the white cells called HLA B27 which occurs with markedly high frequency in patients with these conditions. More than ninety percent of patients with *ankylosing spondylitis* have the HLA B27 gene (B27 positive). On the other hand, perhaps only twenty percent of patients with *psoriatic arthritis* will be B27 positive. Approximately eight percent of the Caucasian American population has this marker, but at most twenty percent of those with the marker will develop the symptoms. Some of these people will also develop related diseases. The HLA B27 marker is less common among African Americans, though they can experience a variant of this disease. Among certain Native American tribes, however, as many as 50 percent have the HLA B27 marker. The currently accepted theory is that the genetic predisposition is necessary for the formation of the disease, but a second event, perhaps an infectious disease, is needed to activate the onset of the enthesopathy.

Ankylosing spondylitis is not a discovery of modern science; traces of it can be found in skeletons dating back to 3000 B.C. The terms come from Greek, where "ankylosing" refers to stiffening or fusing and "spondylos" means backbone. "Itis," as we have noted before, refers to the inflammation that promotes the development of the new bone formation. Unlike many other forms of arthritis, this disease occurs more often in men—two to three times more frequently, in fact. The onset of symptoms before puberty or after the age of 50 is rare. Unfortunately, the disease is rarely diagnosed in a timely manner; often, only after the full-blown picture of stooped posture and bony fusion has emerged, following years of severe back, neck, and leg pain, is the diagnosis reached. The early symptoms are insidious. The typical complaint is of aching in the low back, perhaps with some accompanying pain in the hips or feet. Pain is worse after resting and often is relieved with exercise. Pain and tenderness may localize to the sacroiliac joints (the junction of the spine and the bony pelvis). At times, the pain will radiate into the legs, as in *sciatica.* The patient may have inflammation of different joints, including the hips, knees, ankles, and shoulders.

Curiously, as the joints undergo fusion, the pain often lessens and resolves. In other words, the pain seems to persist only as long as the inflammation is active and the joints are capable of movement.

Ankylosis is not restricted to the vertebrae. In some   instances, it

149

may involve the chest wall, and cause the patient difficulty in taking in a full breath. This can be a highly significant symptom and should be evaluated immediately.

Nor is ankylosis restricted to isolated areas of the body. A small number of patients will develop general systemic problems, including fatigue, weight loss, loss of appetite, and low grade fevers. Some will have an associated inflammation of the eye called *iritis,* while others may develop heart problems, most typically involving inflammation of the aorta, the major blood vessel leading from the heart. In other cases, the lungs may become involved with a scarring or thickening called fibrosis.

Clinically, the diagnosis is based on the presence of *bilateral sacroilitis* (inflammation of the junction between the spine and the bony pelvis) and low back disease, with limited movement of the lumbar spine in all directions. Patients will complain of stiffness, back pain, and pain in the buttocks. The increasing limitation of movement can be measured, as can the decrease of chest expansion. While little change may be seen early, patients with ankylosing spondylitis may eventually develop the characteristic X-ray findings. The sacroiliac joints and much of the spine may fuse into solid bone and resemble a bamboo tree, hence the term "bamboo spine." Some patients do not go on to develop these x-ray findings. This is called non-radiographic axial spondyloarthritis. Magnetic resonance imaging (MRI) has been shown to detect change in the spine and sacroiliac joints much earlier than standard x-rays.

For patients with advanced disease, trauma of any kind can cause severe problems. Lack of mobility tends to make the individual more prone to falls, the rigid spine literally breaking, and causing severe local pain.

Unfortunately, the proper diagnosis of the disease is often delayed, and this delay can have a telling effect on what will become of the patient. Since the onset is slow and insidious, the symptoms are generally misinterpreted as local disease, low back strain, or disc disease. By the time the disease is recognized, the patient has already undergone significant loss of movement. When the disease is diagnosed early, the patient can begin a course of exercise and physical therapy that will enable him or her to maximize movement, ameliorate symptoms, and avoid deformity. Medication may have a powerful impact on this disease particularly when started early in the course of the illness.

Reactive arthritis is another type of enthesopathy and involves the inflammation of either the urethra, the tube from the bladder to the outside *(urethritis)*, the cervix *(cervicitis)*, the eye *(conjunctivitis)*, and arthritis. Many patients with this disease are B27 positive and have a history of venereal or dysenteric infection. Often, the inciting infection appears to be caused by the bacteria Shigella or Yersinia, though other agents, including Chlamydia and Mycoplasma, have been implicated. It may be more severe in those patients who are HIV positive.

With this disease, the patient most frequently complains of discomfort in the legs and ankles. *Achilles tendonitis* frequently causes pain behind the heel, making walking difficult. Arthritis may occur in a single joint, though it more frequently affects multiple joints, usually in a nonsymmetrical or irregular pattern. In such arthritis, the patient may experience not so much inflammation as severe tenderness around the affected joints, with much swelling. The knees are the most frequently involved joints, though *heel spurs* and inflammation of the soft tissue of the soles *(plantar fasciitis)* are also common.

Also, one patient in five with reactive arthritis will develop inflammation of the spine *(spondylitis)* or sacroiliac joints. Some patients develop sausage-shaped swelling in the finger and toes from a diffuse inflammation of the soft tissues.

Reactive arthritis is sometimes accompanied by systemic complications, most notably fever, weight loss, and skin manifestations. A scaly rash with pustules may occur on the soles or the palms, while the nails of the hands may be involved with

151

psoriasis-like changes. Redness and ulceration called *circinate balanitis* may occur on the head of the penis. Painless but recurrent ulcerations may also be found in the mouth. Eye involvement is also possible, with *conjunctivitis,* pus-like discharge, and eye discomfort upon looking at light. More severe eye inflammation, called *iritis,* may also develop, possibly causing permanent damage and even blindness.

Reactive arthritis is presently thought to be a common cause of arthritis in the one or two lower body joints in sexually active young men, occurring 20 times more frequently in men than women. Some investigators feel that this discrepancy is the result of under-reporting in women, as the diagnosis of cervicitis and urethritis in women may be difficult to make. The diagnosis is also frequently missed because the classic symptoms do not always occur simultaneously.

In general, this disease is self-limited with spontaneous improvement. Research now indicates that it persists in at 15 to 20 percent of patients. While its onset appears to be the result of infection, antibiotic treatment has not proven effective. It seems, rather, that the infection triggers the arthritis (reactive arthritis). Nonsteroidal anti-inflammatory drugs provide the standard treatment, but stronger anti-inflammatory medication may be necessary. Active physical and occupational therapy is recommended.

Psoriatic arthritis, another enthesopathy, was once thought to be related to rheumatoid arthritis, perhaps because of the similar deformities produced in both conditions. However, significant differences between the two diseases make the distinction possible in most cases. Between 14 to 30 percent of patients suffering from *psoriasis,* a skin disease, will develop psoriatic arthritis. The arthritis usually occurs after the skin manifestations appear but may precede the skin disease. The disease affects men and women equally, appearing in the 20s and 30s, often suddenly.

Several forms of psoriatic arthritis typically exist. Most common is the development of the disease in a few joints. There may be sausage-like swelling in the hands or feet, for example. The sudden appearance may lead the physician to confuse it with gout, but there are none of the uric acid crystals present in the joint fluid. Spine and sacroiliac joint involvement may occur. The involvement of the distal (end) joint of the fingers, accompanied by changes of the nail also may occur. Other joints involved include the wrist, elbows, knees, and ankles.

Finally, the occurrence of *arthritis mutilans* is probably the most infrequent but also the most debilitating form of the disease. In this form, the obliteration of the joint causes a shortening of the fingers similar to the closing of a telescope.

Since psoriatic arthritis may either mimic or even occur simultaneously with other types of arthritis, the diagnosis may be difficult, though not impossible. Obviously, one helpful factor is the presence of psoriasis, though this may occur after the development of the arthritis. Lab tests usually show an elevated sedimentation rate during flares of the disease, but this is not a specific finding. *Hyperuricemia* (elevated uric acid levels) commonly occurs during periods of flare of the skin disease and may be associated with concurrent gouty flares. Rheumatoid factor, fairly common in the blood in rheumatoid arthritis, is usually absent in psoriatic arthritis.

Imaging procedures such as magnetic resonance imaging and diagnostic ultrasound can be employed as diagnostic tools early on. With advanced disease, distinctive patterns of destruction on x-ray occur.

Treatment includes controlling the associated skin disease. For a few patients, arthritis flares and skin manifestations are clearly linked, though in many cases they appear to be independent of one another. The arthritis is usually managed with nonsteroidal anti-inflammatory drugs and local injections of corticosteroids. Disease modifying antirheumatic drugs, including methotrexate, sulfasalazine, and leflunomide have been used with some success. Biologic agents have been extremely successful in disease control. These include drugs with more specific effects on the immune abnormalities unique to psoriatic arthritis. An even newer non-biologic agent, apremilast (Otezla®), has already shown beneficial effects on this disease in some cases. Physical and occupational therapy are essential for the maintenance of movement, though reconstructive surgery may also become an important option, especially in the severely mutilating forms of the disease.

Another form of enthesopathy is associated with inflammatory bowel diseases, including *ulcerative colitis* and *Crohn's disease (regional ileitis)*. It may also be associated with long-term effects of bypass bowel surgery. Variably named, we will call it simply **enteropathic arthritis**. Often, such arthritis—typically involving the spine or extremity joints—will occur in a patient with an inflammatory bowel disease. The arthritis is felt to be due to bacteria whose proteins cross into the bloodstream through the inflamed and disrupted bowel. Such a scenario is suspected because the arthritis usually comes after the bowel symptoms begin. Usually, the arthritis in such cases involves the large joints and is asymmetric, most commonly attacking the legs. These attacks are usually self-limiting and occur only during a flare of the bowel disease. The joint involvement in such cases is not erosive, so when destructive changes occur, they suggest the presence of other forms of arthritis.

Inflammatory bowel diseases may also be accompanied by a variety of systemic manifestations. The patient may suffer skin involvement, in the form of *erythema nodosum* (painful nodules typically situated in the shins), *aphthous ulcers* (shallow erosions in the mouth or genital area), or *pyoderma gangrenosum* (deep ulcers on the shins). Patients sometimes suffer inflammation of the eye with the inflammatory bowel diseases.

In inflammatory bowel disease, spine involvement may be similar to ankylosing spondylitis, with the HLA B27 gene possibly present. More frequently, however, the arthritis tends to involve the extremities, particularly the knees and ankles.

Treatment of the arthritis is often best accomplished by controlling the bowel inflammation. The arthritis may subside fully for long periods of time when the inflammatory bowel disease itself is under control, even when this is accomplished by removal of the colon. Local steroid injections can help. Treatment of the spinal disease is more difficult. While nonsteroidal anti-inflammatory drugs are frequently used, the side effects, especially bleeding, are more pronounced. Often, sulfasalazine is used in the control of bowel disease, and this has the added benefit of improving the arthritic manifestations as well.

Intestinal bypass surgery, once frequently performed for obesity, is associated with an increased incidence of an arthritis that does not destroy joints but seems to jump from joint to joint. Often, a rash will occur prior to the development of joint symptoms. A red rash may become raised and develop blisters. It is currently believed that bacteria and bacterial proteins accumulate in a blind loop of bowel and do not pass outwardly, so the body responds to these foreign protein antigens by producing increased antibodies. The resultant arthritis in these cases is possibly an immune-mediated phenomenon started by the presence of the bacterial proteins. Treatment with oral antibiotics often helps alleviate the symptoms. The best treatment is to reverse the surgery and eliminate the blind loop.

Whipple's disease is an unusual multisystem disease that clinically has manifestations of arthritis, diarrhea with increased excretion of fats, enlarged lymph nodes, elevated white and platelet counts, fever, and weight loss. Neurologic manifestations commonly occur and vary from burning, tingling, and numbness to brain damage. Arthritis occurs in seventy-five percent of patients with Whipple's disease and often precedes the other symptoms by months and even years. The arthritis usually involves the legs, shoulders, wrists, and, in some cases, the spine. There appears to be a slight increase in HLA B27 positivity. The important diagnostic feature is the presence of specific microscopic inclusion bodies on bowel biopsy. Without treatment, the disease is apparently almost uniformly fatal; in the main, antibiotic treatment is quite effective.

In this chapter, we have attempted to give an overview of the CORE diseases, the identification of their symptoms, and the variety of treatments that are available to victims of these diseases. As we have seen, arthritis can be far more complicated—and, in some cases, far more dangerous—than a pain in the elbow or the knee. And as we note in this chapter, the sooner an individual seeks treatment, the better the overall prognosis is, not just in terms of maintaining movement and personal independence, but in maintaining the very quality of life.

Up to this point, we have considered the symptoms and diagnosis of arthritis and CORE diseases. These are not the only diseases that cause pain in the musculoskeletal system that might be perceived in the least way as arthritis.

In this chapter, we will examine diseases that share the ability to manifest pain in parts of the body other than their site of origin. We have seen such a thing already with *reactive arthritis,* for example, which can manifest on the skin as well as in the gastrointestinal tract. But there are more common diseases and problems that can lead to arthritis-like pain. *Elevated cholesterol* can cause arthritic manifestations. *Carpal tunnel syndrome,* which occurs as the result of compression of the median nerve at the wrist, can be felt in the elbow and the shoulder as well.

Whatever the pain you suffer, it is vital that your doctor examines you. We know it isn't the first time you've read this message in this book, but take comfort; it won't be the last, either. As we saw with the CORE diseases, what you think of as your "arthritis" may actually be a serious, systemic disease that can cause damage to your heart, lungs, and brain as well as your elbow or foot. Remember: When you experience pain, your body is trying to tell you something. It is your responsibility to yourself to do something about it.

Peripheral Neuropathy

Peripheral neuropathy is a condition in which the tiny nerves in the skin function abnormally. This usually occurs in the hands and feet but may also involve the lower legs and thighs. The patient may develop tingling, numbness, burning, or prickling in the affected area. Some patients describe shooting pains, a band-like sensation, or extreme sensitivity to even the most gentle touch. Pain is usually worse at night and may be aggravated by temperature changes.

It is not yet clearly understood what causes these nerves to function in this manner, but many conditions can lead to this problem. *Rheumatoid arthritis; connective tissue diseases* (particularly *lupus* and *Sjögren's syndrome)-, diabetes mellitus; alcoholism; liver disease; kidney disease; thyroid disease; deficiencies in vitamins Bl, B6, and B12; porphyria; cancer; syphilis;* and *Lyme disease*— all may be associated with peripheral neuropathy.

Peripheral neuropathy may also result from the use of certain drugs or medications, including sulfa drugs, phenytoin, nitrofurantoin, isoniazid, metronidazole, excessive vitamin B6, certain drugs for chemotherapy, and many other medications. Finally, exposure to various poisons for short or long periods may bring on peripheral neuropathy. These include arsenic, mercury, carbon monoxide, and certain industrial poisons.

Even with the wide range of possible causes, sometimes the cause of a peripheral neuropathy cannot be found. The condition then is described as being "idiopathic" in origin.

The cornerstone of treatment is to identify the cause of the condition where possible and address that. For instance, if vitamin B12 levels are low due to poor absorption (a condition that can lead to *pernicious anemia),* monthly vitamin B12 injections can easily correct the problem.

However, even when the cause is known, it is sometimes difficult to treat peripheral neuropathy. A number of medications may be useful in relieving the symptoms of the condition, including medications used to treat depression as well as medications that have proven useful in treating epileptic seizures. Some patients describe temporary improvement with the use of mineral ice or support stockings. Electrical stimulation units and analgesic-type balms can sometimes alleviate the discomfort of peripheral neuropathy.

Entrapment Neuropathy

This term really applies to a whole family of afflictions. What they have in common is the way in which the nerve, as it travels through a protective tunnel, is pinched somewhere along its path. The resultant conditions can range from discomforting to disabling. Fortunately, they are generally amenable to traditional treatment modalities.

Carpal Tunnel Syndrome

The carpal tunnel is an actual tunnel in the wrist through which the median nerve passes on its way to the thumb, index finger, middle finger, and the inner half of the ring finger. The tunnel is made up of bony walls and ligaments. The median nerve is subject to damage, due to compression within the tunnel itself. This may be due to inflammation of adjacent structures within the tunnel such as occurs in rheumatoid arthritis and some other inflammatory conditions. The nerve may also suffer direct damage through prolonged or repetitive bending of the wrist or through structural abnormalities that press directly upon the nerve.

When the median nerve is damaged within the carpal tunnel, the patient may experience discomfort in the thumb, index finger, middle finger, and the inner half of the ring finger, even though only one or two of the fingers may actually be involved. Eventually, the hand grip becomes weak, and discomfort radiates through the forearm to the upper arm and even to the shoulder and the neck. The patient often feels that there is a "circulation problem" and often tries to "shake it out" of the hand. Even normal activities such as holding a steering wheel or sleeping may bend the wrist, aggravating carpal tunnel symptoms, and any occupation that involves prolonged or repetitive bending of the wrist can bring on the syndrome.

Swelling within the carpal tunnel itself may occur with *pregnancy, rheumatoid arthritis, enthesopsthies, lupus, gout, pseudogout, tuberculosis,* and *hypothyroidism.* Such swelling puts pressure on the median nerve, causing the symptoms mentioned earlier. Carpal tunnel syndrome may also result from certain structural problems—*bony spurs,* for example, or *ganglia*—that press upon the nerve in the carpal tunnel.

Finally, *vitamin* B6 *deficiency* and *diabetes mellitus* may both damage the median nerve, producing symptoms identical to those of carpal tunnel syndrome.

The condition is diagnosed by physical examination. The nerve is intentionally irritated by either direct tapping on the wrist near the palm or by holding the wrist in a fully bent position for at least 20 seconds. Such actions may reproduce symptoms by aggravating the already irritated median nerve.

Special nerve tests called "nerve conduction velocities" can measure the decreased speed of electrical impulses moving through the injured nerve.

Another way to diagnose median nerve compression in the carpal tunnel is by examining the nerve under ultrasound. Compressed nerves tend to swell proximal to (right before) the constriction. The ultrasound exam will demonstrate this and precisely measure the enlargement. The accuracy of diagnosis rivals that of nerve tests.

Given the broad range of possible causes, it is very important to diligently search for the underlying cause of the carpal tunnel syndrome. Treatment and prevention of recurrence must be based upon thorough understanding of the original cause.

Carpal tunnel syndrome itself is quite treatable. The wrist can be splinted into a "bent-up" position to decrease pressure on the median nerve. A cortisone injection into the wrist may alleviate swelling and pressure within the carpal tunnel. And if necessary, a relatively simple surgical procedure (called a "carpal tunnel release") can be performed to alleviate the pressure within the carpal tunnel. Alternatively, minimally invasive release of the compressed nerve can be accomplished under ultrasound guidance. Recently, an ultrasound-guided thread carpal tunnel release technique has been described.

Ulnar Nerve Compression at the Wrist

The ulnar nerve travels through a tunnel at the wrist called the ulnar tunnel or "Guyon's canal" as it passes into the outside aspect of the ring finger and to the small finger. This is similar to the path followed by the median nerve in the carpal tunnel. And like the median nerve in the carpal tunnel, the ulnar nerve in Guyon's canal may be compressed by inflammation, structural abnormalities, or repetitive bending of the wrist. When this occurs, the individual may feel numbness, tingling, burning, or even weakness in the small finger and the outside aspect of the ring finger. Occasionally, discomfort and pain may travel up the forearm. Both the diagnostic measures and the treatment program for ulnar nerve compression are similar as those for carpal tunnel syndrome.

Cubital Tunnel Syndrome
(Ulnar Nerve Compression at the Elbow)

The ulnar nerve passes through the inside aspect of the elbow on its way to the hand. When pressure is exerted on the ulnar nerve at the elbow, you can get that uncomfortable sensation that is so often— and so wrongly— described as "hitting the funny bone." This is actually irritation of the ulnar nerve.

If the inner aspect of the elbow is injured or inflamed, or if for mechanical reasons the ulnar nerve slips in and out of its groove, thereby becoming irritated, you can develop numbness, tingling, and burning in the outer side of the ring finger and throughout the small finger. The inner aspect of the forearm may also be affected, becoming uncomfortable and tender. The hand, under such circumstances, can become clumsy and the fingers weak.

Other possible causes of ulnar nerve difficulty at the elbow include compression of this area during anesthesia, prolonged periods of resting

161

or leaning on the elbows in an armchair or wheelchair, breaks or fractures of the elbow, and arthritis.

There are various ways to diagnose the condition. If the patient rests the forearm on the head for one minute, he or she will feel burning, tingling, and/or numbness in the forearm and possibly the hand as well. The condition can also be diagnosed easily by an electrical study showing that the electrical impulses through the nerve slow down at the elbow.

Treatment of the underlying cause and avoiding pressure on the inner elbow is often effective. Another treatment modality -ultrasound-guided hydrodissection of the ulnar nerve - may be curative; however, some patients may require surgical release on the ulnar nerve at the elbow for complete relief.

Radial Nerve Palsy

The radial nerve travels down the forearm to the wrist and to the top part of the thumb, the index, and the middle fingers. It may be compressed by the use of crutches or leaning the arm over the back of a chair for a long period of time. In medicinal folklore, this is called "Saturday night palsy." In a similar vein, there is "bridegroom palsy," in which the radial nerve is compresses against the upper part of the arm when the bridegroom falls asleep with his bride's head nestled against his upper arm. When the radial nerve is irritated or damaged, a person can feel numbness, tingling, or increased sensitivity at the top of the thumb, index, and middle fingers as well as on the outside aspect of the forearm. There may even be weakness of the upper arm. The wrist tends to be weak and develops "wrist drop" in which it becomes difficult to bend the hand backwards toward the forearm. Electrical nerve studies are helpful in evaluating this problem.

Thoracic Outlet Syndrome

On each side of the neck is a group of nerves, an artery, and a vein which travels near the collarbone (clavicle) and then down the arm into the hand. This group is called a "neurovascular bundle," and it may be compressed against the collar bone by a neck muscle, an extra rib, or abnormal bone. The condition is usually experienced as numbness, tingling, and burning from the neck down to the arm and hand. Movement of the head and arm in certain positions may aggravate the discomfort. This general condition may be confused with a pinched nerve in the neck.

Pressure upon the neurovascular bundle can be alleviated by treatment aimed at relaxing the tension in the muscle compressing the bundle. Occasionally, surgery is required to relieve the compressive force on the group of nerves and blood vessels.

Meralgia Paresthetica

The lateral femoral cutaneous nerve is a skin nerve that branches from the larger femoral nerve travelling into the thigh from the low back. This skin nerve travels to the upper front and outer aspect of the upper thigh.

The patient may feel constant or intermittent burning in this area, along with increased sensitivity and/or numbness. Standing or walking for a long period of time may produce these symptoms as may certain movements of the thigh. Sitting, on the other hand, may alleviate the discomfort.

The lateral femoral cutaneous nerve may be directly affected by diabetes; however, the most common cause of injury to this nerve is pressure on the nerve as it reaches the skin, resulting from either pressure due to increased weight (such as with pregnancy or a recent weight gain) or the use of a tight binder or corset over the groin area. Legs that are unequal in length or injury to the thigh or groin area may also produce this condition.

Treatment is generally directed at correcting the underlying causes of the problem. Ultrasound guided glucocorticoid injection may help eliminate symptoms.

Tarsal Tunnel Syndrome

The tibial nerve travels down the lower leg to the inner aspect of the ankle and down into the heel. Compression of this nerve may occur in the tarsal tunnel, which is located on the inside aspect of the ankle. This situation is similar to what occurs with median nerve compression in the carpal tunnel in the wrist (see *carpal tunnel syndrome* above). Injury to the foot, occupational wear-and-tear, and various inflammatory conditions may cause pressure on the nerve. Numbness, tingling, and/or burning of the bottom of the heel, the sole of the foot, and the inner aspect of the ankle may occur. The discomfort may be particularly severe at night. An electrical nerve test may help to define the problem more precisely. Treatment may involve injections of the affected area or the prescription of corrective shoes. Ultrasound-guided needle release has been effective in some cases. Surgical release of pressure upon this nerve, however, may be the only effective treatment in some cases.

Tendinopathy, Tendonitis, Tenosynovitis

The tendon is a firm, fibrous tissue. Attached to the bones and muscles, its function is to serve as the pulleys of the muscles, allowing the muscles to exert their force on the bones.

> *Tendinopathy* is simply disease of the tendon.
> *Tendinitis* is acute tendon injury accompanied by inflammation.

The tendon is surrounded by a sheath. This tendon sheath may produce a fluid similar to joint fluid. The tendon sheath can also become inflamed, irritating and fraying the tendon in certain conditions. The resulting condition is generally called *tenosynovitis* and can be the source of significant discomfort.

Many inflammatory diseases may directly involve the tendon and the tendon sheath, among them *rheumatoid arthritis* and *connective tissue diseases, enthesopathies, crystal diseases,* as well as *sarcoidosis* and *gonorrhea.* Injury to the tendon may also result in inflammation, as can pressure due to structural abnormalities *(bony spurs)* and *osteoarthritis.* Repetitive use of a tendon may also result in tendon damage. Quinolone antibiotics, statin medications for cholesterol as well as corticosteroid use are all known to cause tendinopathy.

What follows is a description of the more common types of tendon injuries. This list is not complete, but if used in conjunction with visits to your doctor, it may provide a very good starting point for the identification and treatment of this condition.

Achilles Tendinopathy and Achilles Tendon Rupture

The Achilles tendon is located in the back of the lower leg. It attaches the lower portion of the calf muscle to the area behind the heel. The area can develop inflammation with over-activity, injury, or shoes that press too firmly against the back of the heel.

Other inflammatory conditions may involve the Achilles tendon, including *gout* and other *crystal diseases, rheumatoid arthritis,* and *enthesopathies* (most notably *ankylosing spondylitis* and *Reiter's syndrome).* At the back of the heel, pain, tenderness, and perhaps swelling will develop. Pain occurs particularly when the patient attempts to pull the toes up toward the lower leg.

Treatment consists of rest, correcting any shoe abnormalities, anti-inflammatory medications, and stretching exercises. One treatment that is *not* advised is injection of the Achilles tendon with cortisone as this may lead to the rupture of the tendon.

More recently, the use of ultrasound guided needle tenotomy (peppering the tendon with a small needle) followed by platelet-rich plasma injection has been found to be very effective for treating tendinopathy. Platelet-rich plasma (PRP) is a derivative of a patient's own blood. It is a concentrate containing many platelets which are cells that are rich in growth and healing factors.

The Achilles tendon may rupture or break without a known cause. Upon flipping the top of the foot up toward the shin, for example, a person may hear a snap, followed by pain in the back of the heel and difficulty in walking and standing on the toes. The back of the heel and the lower calf may swell. Patients who have had prior inflammation of the Achilles tendon or who have received cortisone injections in the Achilles tendon are most likely to experience a rupture. Athletic efforts involving the Achilles tendon and direct injury to the tendon itself may also result in a tear.

The ruptured tendon is treated by either immobilizing the leg with a cast or surgery, depending upon the particular case.

Tendinopathy Involving the Knee

The patellar tendon is located at the bottom portion of the patella or kneecap, from where it extends down the short distance to the top of the shin. A common term for *patellar tendinopathy* is "jumper's knee," because this tendon is subject to stress and inflammation among those who jump or run excessively. Pain is located at the bottom of the kneecap.

Treatment consists of anti-inflammatory medications, rest, and the use of ice. Injections of cortisone are not recommended, as these may cause the tendon to rupture. If the tendon ruptures, the patient will experience sharp pain at the bottom of the kneecap and will not be able to straighten the leg. Other possible causes of patellar tendon rupture include injury, repetitive injury from athletic activities, and certain diseases, including *chronic renal failure, rheumatoid arthritis, connective tissue diseases, hyperparathyroidism,* and *gout.* If the tendon ruptures, surgery is often required.

Pain in the back of the knee and toward the outside area may be the result of popliteal *tendinopathy.* This may be due to running, particularly downhill. Rest and anti-inflammatory treatments are usually effective in treating this condition.

Shoulder Tendonitis

The rotator cuff consists of several tendons in proximity to each other whose function is to lift and rotate the upper arm. The rotator cuff tendons either individually or together may become inflamed.

Rotator cuff tendinopathy is often due to the *impingement syndrome.* This occurs when the tendons are pressed up against a bone or ligament, particularly when the arm is lifted up. Repetitive compression of the rotator cuff results initially in inflammation, then in small tears and scar formation. Eventually, bony spurs may develop and further press against the rotator cuff. Rotator cuff tendinopathy may also be associated with a bursitis called a *subacromial bursitis.*

The patient with rotator cuff tendinopathy may have substantial pain upon lifting the arm up. He or she may be engaged in activities that compress the rotator cuff. Barbers and dentists in particular experience rotator cuff tendinopathy due to continual up-lifting of the arms. Pain and tenderness may be exquisite in this area. The patient may have difficulty in dressing him- or herself as well as in finding a comfortable position to sleep at night. X-rays may show calcium deposits either in the tendons or the subacromial bursa.

Treatment generally consists of physical therapy (including hot or cold packs and ultrasound), rest, and anti-inflammatory medications as well as cortisone injections.

Other causes of rotator cuff tendinopathy are those often found with tendinopathy in general, including *crystal diseases, rheumatoid arthritis, connective tissue diseases,* as well as *enthesopathies.* If inflammation and irritation of the rotator cuff persists, eventually a substantial tear may occur in the rotator cuff which can be followed by a complete rupture.

Rotator cuff tear usually occurs when an injury, possibly due to an athletic mishap, coincides with preexisting degenerative and inflammatory changes in the rotator cuff. The rotator cuff may tear without prior disease in the area after a fracture or break of the upper arm or dislocation of the shoulder itself. A rotator cuff tear may be quite small or large, complete or partial. The individual may feel pain and weakness upon lifting the arm up. The shoulder loses range of motion, eventually resulting in a frozen shoulder *(adhesive capsulitis).*

167

Any process that restricts shoulder movement, including pain in the shoulder, may result in frozen shoulder.

Treatment of a rotator cuff tear depends upon the age of the individual and the severity of the tear. It may be treated conservatively with anti-inflammatory medications, rest, and physical therapy.

As with other tendinopathies, ultrasound guided needle tenotomy (peppering the tendon with a small needle) followed by platelet-rich plasma injection has been found to be very effective as a treatment. Platelet-rich plasma (PRP) is a derivative of a patient's own blood. It is a concentrate containing many platelets which are cells that are rich in growth and healing factors.

Occasionally, surgical repair may be necessary.

Biceps Tendinopathy

The biceps tendon helps attach the biceps muscle to the shoulder. The biceps muscle enables us to bend our elbows forcefully. The biceps tendon may become inflamed by impingement or pressure by a bony structure called the acromion. Other conditions, including *crystal diseases, rheumatoid arthritis, connective tissue diseases,* as well as *enthesopathies* may also contribute to *biceps tendinopathy.* Repetitive movement of the biceps tendon is often the culprit, particularly in association with preexisting rotator cuff inflammation. The pain may be of sudden or slow onset, and is usually located at the upper front part of the upper arm. This area is often tender to pressure under normal circumstances but it becomes extremely tender when the biceps tendon is inflamed.

Treatment consists of anti-inflammatory medications, and rest, as well as moist heat and ultrasound.

Eventually, the biceps tendon may become frayed and rupture suddenly, resulting in a round knot that protrudes from the top of the biceps muscle located on the front of the upper arm. This results in the so-called "Popeye's sign." The patient in such cases will experience severe upper arm pain which subsides over days to weeks. Most people who experience rupture of the biceps tendon function quite well and do not require surgical treatment.

The biceps tendon may pop in and out of its groove, resulting in a "popping" or "snapping" shoulder. The upper front area of the upper arm is tender to moderate pressure. This condition is called *biceps tendon subluxation.*

Elbow Tendinopathy

Both "tennis elbow" and "golfer's elbow" are examples of *elbow tendinopathy.* The tennis elbow, also called *lateral epicondylitis,* is located on the outside aspect of the elbow. It can occur with or without playing tennis but often afflicts people who use their arms excessively. Occasionally, direct injury to the outside of the elbow may result in lateral epicondylitis. The outer aspect of the elbow becomes tender to the touch. The patient experiences pain on shaking hands or in picking up objects in which the palm of the hand faces downward— as in picking up a set of keys, for example.

Treatment consists of rest, heat or ice, and anti-inflammatory medications. Occasionally, injections in the elbow may be helpful. Exercises may also prove effective for both treatment and prevention.

"Golfer's elbow" or *medial epicondylitis* occurs on the inner aspect of the elbow and is less common than tennis elbow. Pain occurs in lifting up objects with the palm facing upward—say scooping up ice cubes by hand. The area is often tender to the touch. The treatment is the same as with tennis elbow. PRP injection using ultrasound guidance can be very effective.

Forearm Tendinopathy

De Quervain's tenosynovitis affects specific tendons on the top side of the thumb. These tendons travels up the forearm and it is here particularly that the inflammation is felt. De Quervain's tenosynovitis occurs frequently from moving the wrist while the thumb is made to pinch. One test for this condition is to make a fist in which the thumb on the affected hand is held within the hand's fingers against the palm. This often causes pain on the top of the thumb, across the wrist, and extending up into the forearm. De Quervain's tenosynovitis, then, causes pain in the forearm, wrist, and hand.

Treatment includes splinting, heat or ice, as well as anti-inflammatory medications. Cortisone injection and occasionally surgery may be required to control this disabling condition.

Hand Tendinopathy

The tendons on the top of the hand (the extensor tendons) help to move the top of the hand backward towards the forearm. The tendons on the palm side of the hand (the flexor tendons) help to bend the palm towards the forearm. Both sets of tendons may become inflamed with the kind of systemic conditions described above—*rheumatoid arthritis, crystal diseases,* and related *connective tissue diseases,* as well as *enthesopathies.* Certain infections, such as *fungus* and *gonorrhea,* may inflame these tendons, as may *sarcoidosis.*

There are tendon pulleys in the palms along the tendons that keep them in place. With excess use, these pulleys may thicken, interfering with the patient's ability to straighten the fingers. When the fingers become locked in such a fashion, they are called "trigger fingers." Such conditions may require injection into either the space between the tendon and the pulley. This is best done under ultrasound guidance. Surgery may also be required.

An important part of treatment is to attempt to identify the underlying causes. The physician should also determine if the hands are used excessively for gripping—such as in a patient who has recently acquired the use of a cane. The grip size of the cane may be enlarged to decrease the effort required to maintain control of the cane. This will in turn decrease the stress upon the tendons in the palm of the hand.

Frozen Shoulder (Adhesive Capsulitis)

The frozen shoulder is a condition in which movement of the shoulder is markedly decreased, often with pain and tenderness. The shoulder capsule is a fibrous soft tissue surrounding the shoulder joint. The capsule thickens and contracts in size with time. A frozen shoulder may result from any condition that results in decreased movement of the shoulder, whether it's an inflammatory condition affecting the shoulder or a stroke. It is termed "idiopathic' if there is no discernable cause detected.

Treatment of a frozen shoulder involves a multipronged attack: aggressive physical therapy, nonsteroidal anti-inflammatory medications, and steroid injections into the shoulder. If this fails, the patient may require manipulation of the shoulder. This procedure is done under general anesthesia. In it, the scar tissue is forcibly torn, allowing for improved movement of the shoulder.

Referred Pain

Referred pain is pain that is "transmitted" or "sent" from one area of the body to another. This often occurs in conjunction with nerve problems in which a damaged or irritated nerve sends signals to the brain that are, essentially, misinterpreted by the brain. For example, when a person loses a limb—a leg in an accident, for instance—the irritated nerve remaining in the stump sends signals to the brain which the brain may interpret as pain in the foot. This is called *phantom limb pain*. It is possible, without losing an extremity, to feel pain in parts of the body in which there is no problem.

A very common example of referred pain is *sciatica*. Sciatica usually results from a pinching or irritation of nerve roots in the low back. With sciatica, you may feel pain, numbness, and tingling down the back of the thigh as well as in areas of the lower leg and the foot. You also may feel weakness. The actual cause of the problem, however, can be found in the low back, where the nerve roots emerge from the spinal cord to form the sciatic nerve. The nerve roots or a single root may be pressed upon or pinched by protruding discs or by bony spurs in addition to other structural abnormalities. Sometimes the low back discomfort is minimal and the greatest area of discomfort is the leg. Similar referred pain may occur in the low back but at a slightly higher level where the nerve roots emerge to form the femoral nerve. The specific areas of numbness, tingling, burning, pain, and weakness are described in more detail in the sections on *sciatica* and *femoral neuropathy* later in this chapter.

Arthritic change of the sacroiliac joints may cause pain to radiate into the groin and inner aspect of the thigh. Pain may be felt at the lateral upper thigh as well as the low back. Treatment, in the form of physical therapy, is directed at the sacroiliac joint. (Please see *Sacroiliac joint syndrome* in this chapter.)

Carpal tunnel syndrome, described elsewhere in this chapter, is another example of referred pain. Although the problem resides in the wrist, where the median nerve has been either irritated or compressed, the nerve is sending signals back to the brain describing pain in the forearm, upper arm, shoulder, hand, and even neck. Effective treatment of the nerve at the wrist should stop the related discomfort in all areas. If a nerve is pinched in the neck and wrist simultaneously, treatment of the wrist alone will not suffice to improve the discomfort down the arm. In such instances, called a *double crush injury,* treatment, to be successful, must focus upon both areas of nerve injury.

Pain in the shoulder and especially in the shoulder blade is often the result of problems remote from the shoulder itself. For many years, for example, it has been known that gallbladder pain can be felt at the tip of the shoulder blade in the upper back. The diaphragm, a large muscle separating the chest cavity from the abdominal cavity, moves downward, causing a partial vacuum and allowing air to rush into the lungs. There is a connection between the nerves supplying the diaphragm and the shoulder blade.

When there is irritation of the diaphragm or the lining of the lung over the diaphragm (diaphragmatic pleura), pain can often be felt at the tip of the shoulder blade, particularly when the diaphragmatic pleura is stretched, as in taking a deep breath. Consequently, problems with the gallbladder, the liver, and the diaphragmatic pleura itself may cause pain in the shoulder blade.

Likewise, chest tumors, if located near the nerve that passes around the shoulder blade, may cause pain at the tip of the shoulder blade. Any evidence of shoulder blade discomfort, then, is a symptom that warrants careful evaluation of both the shoulder blade itself as well as the chest and abdominal cavities.

The pain from a diseased gallbladder may be felt in the upper back, not only at the tip of the shoulder blade. Again, the pain is referred through nerve fibers that are particularly sensitive when the patient takes a deep breath or when pressure is applied to the right upper abdomen under the rib cage pressing the already irritated gallbladder.

The lesson to remember: If you experience a discomfort in your upper back that increases when you take a deep breath, you should be evaluated for a variety of possible problems including gallbladder disease and lung conditions.

Just as a nerve root may be pinched in the low back, the nerve roots in the neck may also become pinched and irritated, either by disc protrusion or bony disease. Such conditions result in neck pain as well as pain in the shoulder, upper arm, elbow, forearm, wrist, and hand. This may be accompanied by numbness, tingling, burning, or weakness. Much of the pain may feel distant from the neck—in the hand or the wrist, for example— though such conditions are usually accompanied by significant neck discomfort.

As a result, when evaluating the pain in the hand, arm, or shoulder, one should take into account the possibility of a pinched nerve in the neck—otherwise called cervical radiculopathy, which is described in greater detail elsewhere in the chapter.

Bursitis

A bursa is a small sac that normally contains a small amount of fluid. The bursa acts as a cushion, separating tendons and muscles from other muscles or from bone, and decreasing friction among the components of the musculoskeletal system. Along with all the damaging things that can happen to muscles, tendons, and bones, the bursa itself may be subject to inflammation from any one of a number of different causes. Repetitive movement of the affected joint and tendons, inflammatory conditions like *rheumatoid arthritis,* the crystal *diseases,* infections within the bursa itself, direct irritation from bony spurs and other growths, excessive use—any and all of these factors may lead to bursitis. The specific symptoms of the bursitis depend on the joint involved and the location of the inflamed bursa.

Knee Bursitis

The knee, a complicated joint, has several bursae, any of which can become inflamed.

The anserine bursa is located in the front of the knee on the inner aspect, approximately one inch below the kneecap. When irritated or inflamed, it may cause severe pain, particularly when a person gets up from a chair or goes upstairs.

Anserine bursitis often occurs in middle-aged women who keep their knees together when wearing a dress and who use the right foot for pressing both the gas and the brake pedals when driving. Treatment is rest and anti-inflammatory medications. This condition often requires a cortisone injection to resolve the problem completely.

The prepatellar bursa is located over the kneecap. When it becomes inflamed, the person experiences pain and swelling over the kneecap, though the pain may extend slightly below the knee as well. Often called *housemaid's* or *clergyman's knee,* this condition affects people who are frequently on their knees for prolonged periods of time. Treatment should be directed to the underlying cause. Rest and cortisone injections may help, but if the bursa becomes infected, withdrawing the infected matter from the bursa and treating the patient with antibiotics is the best course of action.

Thigh and Buttock Bursitis

The greater trochanter is a bony protuberance located at the upper outer aspect of the thigh. Over this area are three tendons, each with a bursa beneath them. Any of these bursae they become inflamed and produce localized pain; however, the pain may move either down the lateral aspect of the thigh or diffusely through the entire thigh and hip region. The patient may feel pain when walking or lying down on the affected side. The pain may imitate *sciatica* by moving down the entire lateral aspect of the thigh. The upper aspect of the thigh is locally tender to pressure, but the entire outer aspect of the thigh may also be tender. Occasionally on X-ray, we may see calcification within the bursa itself. Arthritis of the hip and spine as well as unequal leg lengths and back curvature may lead to inflammation of the trochanteric bursae. To make matters more complicated, the overlying tendons may have tendinopathy such as tears that may be the true cause of the pain. Since the pain may be coming from one of three tendons or one of three bursae (or a combination) it is important to precisely delineate the cause with an ultrasound or MRI examination.

Treatment of a trochanteric area bursitis includes anti-inflammatory medications and weight loss. However, the mainstay of treatment is an injection of cortisone directly into the bursa, though surgery may be necessary to treat a chronically inflamed trochanteric bursa. These injections should be done under ultrasound guidance to avoid injecting and damaging the tendons.

Treatment of a trochanteric area tendinopathy may also include anti-inflammatory medication as well as physical therapy but sometimes requires more sophisticated techniques such as tendon fenestration with or without injection of platelet rich plasma to help repair the tendon, all done under ultrasound guidance. Again, corticosteroid injection into the injured tendons will likely make matters worse.

The ischial bursa is located at the undersurface of the pelvis on both sides of the buttock, where the bottom makes contact with the surface upon which a person is sitting. This bursa can become inflamed by prolonged sitting—*weaver's bottom* or *ischial bursitis*. With this condition, pain can be severe when sitting or lying down. Pain may also move down the back of the thigh, imitating *sciatica*. The area is very tender to direct pressure.

Treatment involves using a cushion as well as a direct injection of cortisone into the affected bursa, again, best done using a guidance modality to avoid damaging nerves.

Shoulder and Upper Arm Bursitis

The subacromial bursa helps separate the tendons of the rotator cuff from overlying muscle and bone. The subacromial bursa is at the upper outermost portion of the shoulder and at the very top of the upper arm. It leads downward to the subdeltoid bursa, which lies in the upper third of the outermost aspect of the upper arm.

The subacromial bursa may become inflamed as a result of the *impingement syndrome.* The impingement is caused by bone or ligament in the coracoacromial arch. This bursa may also be inflamed with conditions such as *rheumatoid arthritis, connective tissue disease,* the *crystal arthropathies,* overuse, and *bony spur formation* pressing upon the bursa and tendons.

As noted before, certain professions—hairdressing, for example, or dentistry—often lead to bursitis in the shoulder and upper arm because of prolonged periods of raising the arms, causing pressure against the bursa and the tendons.

The pain of *subacromial bursitis* is felt directly in the shoulder and the region of the outer upper arm. Lifting up the arm aggravates the pain. Direct injection of cortisone into the bursa can be effective in alleviating the pain. The use of anti-inflammatory medications and rest can also help, though occasionally surgery may be required.

The bursa itself may show calcification on X-ray. Such calcium deposits may "flake off" from time to time, causing crystal fragments to reactivate inflammation of the bursa. Such calcium deposits may have to be removed to ensure long-lasting relief.

Elbow Bursitis

The olecranon bursa is located near the bony part of the elbow where the elbow meets the outside of the forearm. Since this bursa does not connect directly with the elbow joint, inflammation of the bursa does not decrease movement of the elbow itself.

Trauma, either chronic continuous pressure, for example) or acute, may cause inflammation of the bursa. *Rheumatoid arthritis* and *crystal diseases* (such as *gout* or *pseudogout)* may inflame this bursa. Patients undergoing hemodialysis may develop *olecranon bursitis,* perhaps due to *crystal disease.*

The olecranon bursa, because it lies close to the surface of the skin, is easily infected. Bacteria may seed into it as a result of even a minimal trauma. If infected, it can be drained and the patient treated with an antibiotic, which generally, solves the problem.

If no infection is noted, anti-inflammatory medications, relief of direct pressure on the area, and possibly a direct injection of cortisone may be all that is needed to treat this bursitis.

While the discomfort associated with the inflammation of this bursa may be minimal, the elbow can be subject to significant swelling, with sensations of tender pain occurring only on direct pressure.

177

Chondromalacia Patellae

This term describes an abnormality of the cartilage behind the kneecap that results in poor kneecap movement. More modern sources describe this condition as *patellofemoral pain syndrome* or *patellofemoral dysfunction,* characterizing the poor movement of the kneecap when the joint is bent and then straightened. The patient experiences pain behind the kneecap as well as a symptom called *crepitus*—the grinding sensation of bone upon bone behind the kneecap.Pain occurs after the patient has been sitting for a prolonged period of time. Activity will provide some relief, though certain actions, such as climbing a set of stairs, will likely cause a sharp pain behind the kneecap.

The syndrome can be caused by any one of a number of different problems: direct injury to the kneecap involving the cartilage behind it as well as certain congenital kneecap problems.

In congenital affliction, younger patients may feel pain in both knees. Treatment consists of anti-inflammatory medications, rest, and physical therapy. Surgery is rarely necessary.

Hamstring Tightness

The hamstring muscles are located behind the thighs. The tendon attaches to the lower portion of the back of the pelvis passing behind the knee to insert on the upper portion of the foreleg bones. The hamstring muscles are used to bend the knee. These muscles and tendons may become tight or shortened when a person does not frequently stretch or straighten out the knee. The norm of day-to-day living is too often associated with sitting; rarely do people take a few minutes every day just to stretch the knees.

Tightness in the hamstring may also occur in individuals with knee problems who find that the most comfortable position is with the knee slightly bent. Usually, those who suffer from an inflammation of the knee find some relief with the knee slightly bent, as it lightens pressure within the knee by increasing the volume of the knee. Patients may involuntarily bend the knee in such circumstances, leading to tightened, shortened hamstring muscles and tendons. Eventually, this produces discomfort behind the knee and behind the thigh.

Generally, treatment is directed at identifying and correcting any underlying problem as well as in educating the patient in the most effective and efficient ways of stretching the hamstrings regularly.

Aseptic Necrosis

Aseptic necrosis has various names, including *osteonecrosis, avascular necrosis,* and *ischemic necrosis of the bone.* Essentially, the bone begins to die in the areas affected. Most commonly, aseptic necrosis affects the hip, the shoulder, and the knee. People most likely to suffer from aseptic necrosis are those who have previously fractured a hip, a shoulder or a knee. Attempts to save the native bone and maintain adequate blood flow to the joint are not always successful. How to maintain adequate blood flow with such fractures is not yet fully established.

An increasing number of cases of aseptic necrosis are being associated with chronic cortisone use, whether it is cortisone prescribed to patients for other conditions or produced in excess in the body itself by the adrenal gland in a condition called *Cushing's syndrome.*

Other conditions independent of cortisone use and treatment may predispose an individual to aseptic necrosis. These include *lupus erythematosus, abnormal hemoglobin* such as in *sickle cell anemia, alcoholism,* certain tumors such as *leukemia* and *Hodgkin's disease, gout,* direct injury to the area, inflammation of the arteries or *arteritis, sarcoidosis,* and *Caisson disease ("decompression sickness"* or *"the bends".* Aseptic necrosis may cause severe localized pain in the involved joint. In a far-advanced case, an X-ray will show the disintegrating bone. Early cases may be diagnosed by either bone scan or MRI (magnetic resonance imaging). Surgery is often required to correct the problem.

Jaw and Temporomandibular Joint Pain

The temporomandibular joint is the hinge upon which the jaw moves. Located in the front of the skull, just below each ear, this is every bit as much a joint as a shoulder, say, or a hip; that is, it has a lining of synovium and each joint surface is covered by cartilage. In addition, as with other joints, there is a meniscus or "shock absorber" located within the temporomandibular joint.

Pain in the temporomandibular joint may be localized, or it may be experienced elsewhere around the head—as facial pain, for example, headache, or neck pain. The joint itself may be subject to *osteoarthritis* or such inflammatory diseases as *rheumatoid arthritis* and other *connective tissue diseases.* Even *gout* affects this joint! *Angina,* poor blood flow to the heart, may cause pain to radiate from the chest up to the jaw. Occasionally, anginal discomfort may be felt only in the jaw.

Temporal arteritis, also known as *giant cell arteritis,* is an inflammatory condition affecting the blood vessels, primarily in the head. When this problem begins to manifest, the jaw may become uncomfortable, particularly when chewing or after prolonged talking because the blood flow to this joint decreases as the blood vessels themselves become inflamed. Toothaches, nerve problems such as *tic douloureux, sinus conditions, ear difficulties,* and *disorders of the parotid* (salivary) *glands* may all cause pain in the jaw.

Another common cause of jaw pain is *temporomandibular joint syndrome* or TMJ *syndrome,* which can affect either side or both sides of the jaw. Discomfort is often worse in the morning, due to the unconscious clenching or grinding of the teeth during sleep. Pain may also be aggravated by chewing food. The patient may experience pain in the neck and migraine-type headaches. Pain is further aggravated by mental stress and by dental work, during which the mouth has been held open for a prolonged period of time. With TMJ syndrome, the patient may feel a grinding or clicking sensation in the jaw and, if there is an abnormality of the meniscus of the joint, may experience a feeling of the jaw locking into one position.

Direct injury to the jaw may lead to joint abnormalities or abnormal muscle tension. If the patient's bite is abnormal, for instance, this problem may cause unusual stresses upon the chewing action of the jaw. This in turn may lead to secondary TMJ dysfunction and lead into a cycle of pain, abnormal jaw movement, and continued joint dysfunction.

Abnormal posture of the neck may also affect jaw position, possibly precipitating or exacerbating a TMJ syndrome. Eventually, such abnormal movement of the TMJ joint may result in *secondary osteoarthritis* of the joint itself, which in turn can lead to further damage to the joint and its muscles.

Treatment of TMJ syndrome is usually conservative. The patient is asked to avoid abnormal or prolonged chewing. Local applications of heat and ice are often suggested. Anti-inflammatory medications in conjunction with physical therapy is part of a fairly common treatment plan, while a bite plate for night wearing and the correction of any malocclusions are typical in cases where overbite is evident. Muscle relaxants, antidepressants, and stress management techniques may all be of use in the treatment of this problem. Occasionally, the joint may be injected with cortisone. If that fails, surgery may be required as a last resort, particularly if the meniscus proves to be abnormal in its formation.

Sciatica and Femoral Neuropathy

Many people who have low back pain think that they have "sciatica." At heart, though, true sciatica is the irritation of the nerve roots that form the sciatic nerve. Such irritation may result from a ruptured or herniated disc in the low back that presses upon the nerve roots. The disc is composed of soft tissue and is shaped like a jelly doughnut. Located between the vertebral bodies, the bony building blocks of the spine, these discs are vulnerable to injury through stress (injury to the low back), accident, or such traumas as excessive lifting, particularly when the back has been injured before.

Any one of these can lead to the rupture of a disc. But for sciatica to occur, the disc rupture must be large enough to press upon the nerve root, producing numbness, tingling, burning, and/or pain anywhere along the length of the sciatic nerve. That includes the back of the thigh, down the back and outermost portion of the lower leg, and in the outer aspect of the foot and the sole. The leg may be weakened and the reflexes as tested by your doctor may seem less responsive.

The femoral nerve, which emerges from the spinal cord in the low back somewhat higher than the sciatic nerve, is prone to similar problems. With *femoral neuropathy,* the sensations of tingling, numbness, burning, and/or pain will shift toward the front of the thigh and the inner aspects of the lower leg. Disc rupture is less likely in the femoral nerve root areas, but a car accident or lifting an overly heavy load may still do the damage.

Both the femoral and the sciatic nerve roots may be pressed upon by bony spurs (due to *osteoarthritis)* or other growths. Similarly, any process or condition that affects the sciatic or femoral nerve after it has formed outside the spinal cord may produce "sciatica-like" symptoms.

The specific area of nerve irritation may be delineated by spinal electrical nerve studies and imaging of the spine—most notably magnetic resonance imaging. Sciatica and femoral neuropathy are usually quite treatable with conservative measures; however, surgical treatment is sometimes necessary.

"Pinched Nerve in the Neck"
or Cervical Radiculopathy

The discs, shaped like jelly doughnuts, are comprised of soft tissue and are located between the vertebral bodies or bony building blocks of the spine. Their purpose is to serve as shock absorbers for the spine. However, in certain circumstances— say, a car accident—the neck may be thrown forward and backward in a "whiplash" effect, causing one or more of the discs to herniate or rupture. Soft material emanating from the disc may press on the nerve root, causing numbness, tingling, burning, pain, and/or weakness in the neck, shoulder, upper arm, forearm, and hand. This is called *radiculopathy.* (Radicular refers to the nerve root.)

Such nerve root irritation may also occur from bony spurs resulting from *osteoarthritis.*

Conservative treatment, including physical therapy and traction of the neck is often successful. Electrophysiologic studies of the nerve may help determine exactly where the nerve problem originates.

Herniated or Ruptured Disc

As noted above, the disc is a soft tissue that is not unlike a jelly doughnut: soft inside, firmer outside. Situated between the bony vertebral bodies, the discs confer flexibility to the back and provide shock-absorbing protection for the spine.

A disc may rupture due to weakening of the outer fibers, particularly in the face of sudden stress, such as a car accident or the improper lifting of a heavy load. As with *sciatica,* the soft inner material of the disc may protrude and press on a nerve root and cause irritation and discomfort anywhere and everywhere along the length of the nerve (see *"sciatica* and *femoral neuropathy"* and *"cervical radiculopathy"*)

Other terms for a ruptured or herniated disc include a "slipped disc" and a "protruding disc." The discomfort, location, and severity of the patient's problem are determined by the specific location of the herniated disc along the spine. Bony spurs, due to *osteoarthritis,* may also cause sciatica, femoral neuropathy, and cervical radiculopathy by directly pressing upon nerve roots.

Special electrophysiologic nerve studies help identify specifically where the pinching of the nerve is occurring.

If disc herniation or arthritis spurs press on the spinal cord, a condition called myelopathy can occur. Patients will complain of weakness and their physical exam will show profound abnormalities in strength and reflexes. Myelopathy is a surgical emergency.

Spinal Stenosis

The spinal canal is a bony canal that sheaths the spinal cord. In a normal spinal canal, the spinal cord is uninhibited by the internal walls of the canal. Spinal stenosis refers to the narrowing of the spinal canal, a problem that affects the low back more often than any other area of the spine.

There are numerous causes of spinal stenosis. A developmental abnormality such as a congenitally narrowed spinal canal may lead to the condition. *Paget's disease,* a metabolic disease that leads to abnormal bone regeneration, may also bring on spinal stenosis, as may *bony spurs* brought on by *osteoarthritis. Ruptured or herniated discs* may protrude upon the spinal canal, aggravating or causing spinal stenosis, particularly when the spinal canal is congenitally narrowed or bony spurs are already present. Scar tissue within the spinal canal, particularly after low back surgery, may also contribute to spinal stenosis. Misalignment of the bony vertebrae due to either congenital or traumatic causes may aggravate the situation.

A patient suffering from this condition feels pain moving down from the back into the legs. Other sensations include leg numbness and weakness. These occur particularly with walking and can be alleviated by stopping walking, sitting, or bending forward slightly. When the spine is bent forward, the diameter of the spinal canal increases a little—enough, at least, to lessen the discomfort of the spinal stenosis.

Next time you're at the supermarket, watch for people who are bent forward over their shopping carts. A good number of them will be attempting to alleviate symptoms of spinal stenosis as they move down the aisle. The lower-leg discomfort some people describe as "poor circulation" is, in fact, the manifestation of spinal stenosis in the lower legs, though it does mimic poor blood supply to arteries in the legs.

Spinal stenosis may be diagnosed by CAT scan or magnetic resonance imaging evaluation. This is quite treatable. Generally, surgery has proven so far to be the most effective treatment.

Tailbone Pain

The tailbone or coccyx is located at the very end of the spine. The coccyx may be bruised or broken (fractured) after a fall on the tailbone. The area is usually quite tender. Treatment is generally restricted to using a "doughnut" or ringed seat to take pressure off the tailbone when sitting, and pain medication may be helpful.

Coccydynia simply means tailbone pain. In this situation, there is no clear-cut history of bruising or traumatizing the area. The pain in such cases may be due to a forgotten episode of prior trauma or to sitting on hard surfaces for long periods of time. It is important to make certain that there is no underlying infection and that the pain is not being referred from either a gynecological, intestinal, or low back problem.

Once the diagnosis has been confirmed, treatment is similar to that of a coccyx bruise or fracture—that is, using a ringed seat and avoiding prolonged sitting on firm surfaces. A local injection of cortisone can sometimes be quite helpful for coccydynia.

Hoarseness

Hoarseness is often a sign of underlying conditions quite separate from problems within the throat itself. Naturally, a thorough evaluation of the throat and vocal cords by an ear, nose, and throat doctor is in order if hoarseness has persisted for more than several weeks, but if the condition remains, a variety of possible causes need to be accounted for.

For example, *hypothyroidism* (underactive thyroid) causes hoarseness. Also, reflux of acid into the esophagus may occur when the muscle at the end of the esophagus, or food tube, is less tight than it should be. The acid may reflux all the way up into the back of the throat and cause inflammation there as well as a hoarse voice. *Rheumatoid arthritis* may involve joints within the neck and throat in a condition called *cricoarytenoiditis*. Usually, patients with this problem already have well-documented cases of rheumatoid arthritis and are actively flaring with the disease in other areas of the body.

Another cause of hoarseness is *pericardial effusion*, when fluid accumulates in the sac around the heart. Such fluid accumulation may occur for a number of reasons, but regardless of the cause, there can be hoarseness because the accumulated fluid can involve a nerve in the area that has connections to the voice box. A simple heart evaluation by chest X-ray or better yet by a sound wave test (echocardiogram) may be quite helpful in diagnosing the problem.

Several forms of tumor may include voice hoarseness among their symptomatology. Cancer of the esophagus may involve a nerve that controls the voice box. There may also be metastatic involvement from such a tumor involving the throat—that is, the tumor has spread into the throat. Lung tumors may also spread into the throat area or involve nerves that control the voice box even though these nerves may be somewhat remote from the throat. Obviously, cancer involving the neck may directly impinge upon the voice box itself or a nerve controlling the voice box.

Because of the potentially serious nature of many of the above conditions, we strongly encourage every reader to seek professional help any time hoarseness does not pass quickly.

Wry Neck (Acute Torticollis)

Wry neck usually occurs suddenly, with muscle pain and spasm causing significant discomfort on one side of the neck. There is usually no known injury. A patient may awaken with the neck leaning to one side because of the discomfort. This also may occur after sitting for a long time with the neck in an unusual position or from exposure to cold or damp weather. The involved side is quite tender and movement of the neck is limited.

Torticollis may occur as a reaction to certain medications, including the "anticholinergic" medications, such as the antihistamine class, metoclopramide (used to aid nausea and acid reflux into the esophagus), and certain medications used to treat schizophrenia.

Treatment for wry neck is usually conservative, comprising heat treatment, physical therapy, pain medications, and muscle relaxants. A neck collar can sometimes help. If the wry neck is due to a drug reaction, it may be reversed with the use of another medication called benztropine.

Acute Neck Strain

A neck strain generally occurs with overuse, though tiny tears in the neck muscle may be the result of a sudden jarring movement of the neck (as in a whiplash injury). Neck strains also occur after the neck has been kept in an abnormal position for a prolonged period of time or after overuse. Conservative treatment is usually effective—moist

187

heat, pain medications, and a neck collar.

Neck Sprain (Whiplash)

The victim of whiplash often has a history of an impact bending the head forward, then backward, then forward again. This is what happens in a car accident and is called a *sudden deceleration injury.* The ligaments are sprained or develop tears, and the resultant pain can be quite severe. The patient should be examined for fractures (bone breaks) in the neck as well as dislocations and possible disc ruptures.

Conservative treatment often is effective, and includes the use of a collar, rest, ice, and heat as well as pain medications, muscle relaxants, and anti-inflammatory medications.

Ganglion

A ganglion appears as a lump that can develop on the wrist. It is actually a sac filled with a thick, jelly-like fluid that emerges from a wrist joint or tendon sheath. It may result from injury to the wrist, osteoarthritis, or repetitive bending of the wrist over an extended period. Generally, a ganglion only causes swelling; however, it may cause local pain or give rise to *carpal tunnel syndrome.* The latter occurs when the ganglion becomes large enough to press against the median nerve and exert pressure on the median nerve. A ganglion in a different wrist location may also press upon the ulnar nerve causing compression of that nerve.

Treatment is usually conservative. If the ganglion is small and causes no discomfort, the practice is to ignore it. The age-old remedy is to hit the ganglion with a book- often the family Bible!- though there is no compelling study that suggests this treatment actually works. Another treatment for a ganglion is to insert a needle and remove the fluid before injecting the site with cortisone. Unfortunately, the ganglion tends to recur with this method of treatment. Occasionally, the ganglion may require surgical removal.

Dupuytren's Contracture

A Dupuytren's contracture is a thickening of the fibrous tissue in the palm of the hand. Usually this starts off with small nodules forming in the palm, perhaps in a line, connecting to the ring finger. The small, ring, and middle fingers may all become involved. There is no direct involvement of the nerves, muscles, tendons, or joints. The thickening process in the palm may eventually cause the fingers to contract toward the palm. The progress of this condition varies enormously from one patient to the next. The cause is unknown, but there does seem to be evidence that heredity plays a role. The condition is most common among male whites.

While no specific cause has been found, there is an association between Dupuytren's contracture and liver disease (as occurs with chronic alcoholism) and even epilepsy.

The hand usually remains quite functional; however, if the contracture becomes too severe, local surgery may be needed. Other, more conservative treatment includes heat, physical therapy, and local cortisone injections. More recently, local injection with a medication called collagenase clostridium histolyticum has been successful in dissolving the fibrous tissue.

Costochondritis or Tietze's Syndrome

Costochondritis and Tietze's syndrome are terms used to describe inflammation of the cartilage attaching the ribs to the breast bone (sternum). Other names used to describe the condition are *anterior chest wall syndrome, costosternal syndrome, costochondrodynia, and parasternal chondrodynia.* Although these other terms describe pain in this cartilage, costochondritis (Tietze's syndrome) implies enough inflammation to cause local swelling. Costochondritis may follow an

189

injury or be associated with inflammatory diseases of the cartilage—for example, *relapsing polychondritis.*

Costochondritis affects all age groups, including children. The patient experiences upper frontal chest pain which may be severe and can radiate to the shoulder or arm. Sneezing, coughing, taking a deep breath, bending, lying in bed, or physical exertion may all increase the pain. Touching the area can also be painful. If the lower cartilage is affected, the patient may experience pain in the abdomen.

It is important to separate the chest pain produced by costochondritis or Tietze's syndrome from that produced by the heart or other deep structures in the chest.

Treatment consists of anti-inflammatory medication and often the use of local cortisone injection.

Sternal Tip Syndrome

Sternal tip syndrome is similar to costochondritis in that the cartilage at the lowest portion of the breast bone becomes inflamed and tender to the touch. Other terms for sternal tip syndrome include *hypersensitive xiphoid, cartilage syndrome,* and *xiphoidalgia.* The patient may experience upper abdominal pain, nausea, and vomiting. Local injection of cortisone is often effective in eliminating the discomfort.

Shoulder-Hand Syndrome
(Reflex Sympathetic Dystrophy Syndrome
or Chronic Regional Pain Syndrome)

Shoulder-hand syndrome is also known as reflex sympathetic dystrophy syndrome (RSDS) or, chronic regional pain syndrome (CRPS), and is a poorly understood condition in which an extremity, often the hand and arm, develops severe burning pain with associated swelling and tenderness. It may also involve the leg. The condition is also called *causalgia, reflex neurovascular dystrophy, Sudeck's atrophy,* and *algodystrophy.*

The shoulder-hand syndrome was first noted during the Civil War among soldiers injured in the extremities. Nowadays, it can be seen after joint or spine surgery or injury, or in patients who have had a stroke or a heart attack. It has also been noted among patients using certain medications, including barbiturates and isoniazid.

Keeping a hand or leg at rest for prolonged periods of time seems to increase the tendency toward the condition. It is generally known as shoulder-hand syndrome because the patient experiences pain and swelling in the hand and pain in the shoulder of the involved side.

In addition to severe pain and swelling of the involved extremity, other symptoms include local tenderness, abnormal temperature, and color changes. Bone calcium may decrease in the affected limb.

The exact cause of CRPS is unclear. It is felt that it can be attributed to an abnormal neurologic mechanism in response to an injury. But this theory is only speculative.

The extremity involved with CRPS may eventually become atrophied or withered—an essentially useless hand or foot. Pain may subside, but it may also continue indefinitely.

Diagnosis is based upon the history and physical evaluation as well as X-ray and bone scan evaluation. Treatment consists of physical therapy and a variety of medications. At times, anesthetic blocks of part of the nervous system have proven helpful. Occasionally, patients undergo sympathectomies, the surgical destruction of part of the nervous system called the sympathetic division of the autonomic nervous system.

A critical thing to remember in possible cases of CRPS: early diagnosis and aggressive early treatment are generally far more effective than the frequent failure of treatment in later stages.

Shoulder Periarthritis

The shoulder, as a joint, is surrounded by a soft tissue called the joint capsule. Occasionally, the joint capsule itself becomes inflamed, resulting in shoulder pain and, eventually, *frozen shoulder* due to fibrous adhesions.

Two endocrine diseases that may be associated with shoulder periarthritis are *diabetes mellitus* and *hyperthyroidism* (overactive thyroid gland). It is unclear precisely how these conditions affect the shoulder capsule; but patients with shoulder pain and decreased shoulder movement should be evaluated for both diabetes and hyperthyroidism. Treatment in these cases is directed not only to the shoulder but also to any underlying condition that precipitated the shoulder problem in the first place. Treatment includes shoulder injections, physical therapy and occasional manipulation under anesthesia to break up the adhesions.

Brachial Plexus Injury

The brachial plexus is a group of nerves formed of the nerve roots in the neck as they emerge from the spinal cord. The brachial plexus then goes on to form the nerves traveling into the shoulder, upper arm, forearm, and hand. The brachial plexus is located behind the collarbone close to the neck.

The nerve group may be injured in car accidents, gunshot wounds, and other traumatic events. *Diabetes* may also affect the brachial plexus. The plexus may also become inflamed (a condition called brachial plexitis) from viral infection. Abnormal function of the brachial plexus is called *brachial plexopathy.*

Regardless of the cause of brachial plexus dysfunction, the patient often experiences significant pain in the armpit, shoulder, arm, and hand. Numbness, tingling, and burning may course into the shoulder and down the arm and weakness of the shoulder and arm is common. The scapula or shoulder blade on the affected side may be "winged"— that is, the shoulder blade sticks out directly from the upper back when compared with the unaffected side. Neurologic problems are often the cause of a winged scapula.

Treatment of the brachial plexus injury depends on the underlying condition. When it occurs after a virus, the condition is self-limited and usually improves within a few weeks. Rest, use of an arm sling, and anti-inflammatory medications are the standard course. More permanent injury to the brachial plexus—following a car accident or a gunshot wound, for example—may require a surgical approach; conservative treatment in these circumstances has generally been ineffective.

Raynaud's Phenomenon

Raynaud's phenomenon is caused by reversible spasm in the small arteries of the hands and feet. The artery spasm may be caused by exposure to cold temperature or emotional stress. Following the spasm, there is a characteristic series of color changes from white to blue to red in the fingers or the toes. These changes may be accompanied by pain. Raynaud's phenomenon may occur as an isolated problem—then termed *Raynaud's disease.* This condition is particularly common in young women.

Secondary Raynaud's commonly occurs with many of the *connective tissue diseases,* including *scleroderma, mixed connective tissue disease, lupus, myositis,* and *rheumatoid arthritis.* The Raynaud's phenomenon may actually precede the appearance of one or more of these diseases.

Secondary Raynaud's may also occur with occupational trauma, especially when the individual is subject to repetitive percussion or vibration, as in the use of jackhammers.

Raynaud's may also occur when the blood is thickened by an increased number of red blood cells *(polycythemia)* or increased protein production (such as with a bone marrow tumor called *multiple myeloma)*. Many drugs can induce Raynaud's, including ergots (used for migraine headaches) and beta blockers (used for blood pressure and angina control).

Raynaud's may also be associated with certain chemical exposures, including polyvinyl chloride. Smoking aggravates the condition.

Hamate Hammer Syndrome

This is an occupational hazard that affects workers who use their hands. When the heel of the hand is used to pound things into place (plumbers, electricians, carpenters, auto mechanics), trauma to the ulnar artery can lead to restricted blood flow to the hand. This can cause a Raynaud's like syndrome to develop in that hand. A clue may be the presence of numbness in the fourth and fifth fingers due to associated involvement of the ulnar nerve.

Sarcoidosis

Sarcoidosis (or sarcoid, for short) is an inflammatory disease of unknown cause that can affect almost any part of the body. It typically occurs in young women and may inflame the ankles or knees, as well as the small joints of the hands, wrists, and elbows. In addition, the tendons of the hands and feet may become inflamed with the disease. Sarcoidosis often involves the lymph nodes of the lungs, causing a perceptible enlargement of the nodes when viewed on a chest X-ray. The inflammation can spread to the eye and skin, causing red painful lumps on the shins called *erythema nodosum* ("erythema" means red and "nodosum" means like a nodule). The inflammation may also involve muscles of the arms, legs, and the heart. Other possible organs involved include the spleen, the bone marrow, and the bones.

194

In the blood, some patients with sarcoidosis have an elevated protein called angiotensin converting enzyme (ACE) and some patients have high blood calcium levels.

The arthritis of sarcoidosis may imitate the arthritis of *inflammatory bowel disease, rheumatic fever,* and *rheumatoid arthritis.* Once diagnosed, sarcoidosis is quite treatable with anti-inflammatory medications.

PART THREE:
WHAT CAN I DO?

Up to this point, we have been concentrating on trying to identify the problems—the causes of your suffering, your aches, and your pains. We have even indicated various avenues of treatment your doctor may prescribe to help you feel better, if not completely well.

Still, there are some things that you can do on your own— indeed, there are some things that you will have to do. For example, how aware are you of the foods you eat, the vitamins and minerals you take? Are the medications you are already taking somehow affecting your overall condition in ways that you do not know?

These are important questions. In the next two chapters, we lead you through questions of diet and medications, and how vitamins, minerals, nutrition and drugs affect the way you feel. The next chapter includes charts so you can look up the vitamins, and minerals pertinent to your condition. The following chapter on "Drugs and Discomfort" will help you to find an excellent source for determining if your medications, either by themselves or in concert with each other, are the source of your problem. The better you can identify your condition, the better you'll be to discuss it with your doctor.

Finally, in chapter 12, we address the problem of finding the right doctor. Though self-monitoring is a very important tool in the promotion of better living, there are just far too many things that only a doctor can do. Choosing the right doctor can make an extraordinary difference in your life.

Diet and Illness

The notion that what we eat affects pain and causes arthritis has stirred debate for many years. An extraordinary number of unproven dietary remedies appear in this country each year. Authorities contended for a long time that were was no clear-cut association between food and pain, barring a few notable exceptions, and they asserted that food did not cause or worsen arthritis. Medical research, however, has proven that there is much more of a relationship between food and pain than just heartburn.

Celiac Disease

Over the past ten years the awareness of a condition called celiac disease or *gluten enteropathy* has surged in the media. This condition underscores that foods we eat may profoundly affect our state of health. The patient with celiac disease develops inflammation of the lining of the small bowel upon ingesting gluten, a protein found in wheat. This can lead to diarrhea, weight loss, bloating and poor absorption of nutrients. This disease may exist in a form that does not produce these more severe gastrointestinal manifestations but nevertheless can still lead to many problems. Celiac disease is associated with diabetes and a skin condition called dermatitis herpetiformis. There are reported associations with osteoarthritis, thyroid, liver and kidney disease among others. Only further research and time will tell how true these associations turn out to be.

The disease can be diagnosed by a blood test in most cases. Treatment is avoiding gluten in the diet.

Diet and Gout

One of the best documented associations between food and arthritis is *gout.* Gout occurs when uric acid inflames the soft tissues and joints. Uric acid is one of the byproducts of purine nucleic acids, the building blocks of genetic materials in the body. The greater the level of blood uric acid, the greater the chance of gout. Purines ingested in excess quantity may increase blood uric acid levels which, in turn, may lead to gout. Foods high in purine content include organ meats (kidneys, liver, sweetbreads), anchovies, sardines, mussels, herring, broths, gravies, and fish roe. Other foods containing less but still significant purines include red meats, peas, cauliflower, lentils, yeast, beans, asparagus, mushrooms, spinach, whole grain cereals, fowl, and fish.

Alcohol, including wine and beer, increases uric acid production and inhibits uric acid excretion by the kidney. The result is an increase in blood uric acid level.

Finally, gout may be the result of the ingestion of lead, such as that found in moonshine whiskey. Moonshine in the past was often brewed in automobile radiators which leach out a great deal of lead in the distilling process. The lead causes kidney damage, inhibiting the ability of the organ to excrete uric acid, which in turn leads to gouty episodes.

It should be noted that blood uric acid levels are not only related to gout; they also have a direct correlation with obesity.

Cholesterol, Fat, and Arthritis

Two basic fats in the body are cholesterol and triglycerides, both of which are associated with arteriosclerosis (hardening of the arteries). What is not commonly known is that elevated cholesterol and triglycerides may also cause joint pain, tendon pain, and swelling, thereby creating conditions that look and feel like different forms of arthritis.

Generally, when the level of cholesterol or triglycerides is sufficiently high, the cause is often genetic. However, diet may affect the severity of the pain, by influencing the blood levels of these fatty substances.

Diet and the Immune System

The immune system does battle with what it recognizes as foreign invaders in the body, such as bacteria and viruses. Certain vitamins, particularly vitamin B6, vitamin C, vitamin A, and vitamin E are necessary for the integrity of the immune system. As you will see later in this chapter, both deficiencies *and* excesses of a number of vitamins may prompt significant illness.

Recent studies suggest that decreased immune response occurs with low protein or low saturated fat/low cholesterol diet. With this in mind, researchers in one study attempted to use diet to manipulate the immune system to treat two inflammatory diseases, *lupus* and *rheumatoid arthritis.* In the so-called "fish oil" diet, patients with these diseases fed a diet high in unsaturated fat had improvement of their inflammation. This improvement is believed to have resulted from the lessening of the level of saturated fats which often serve as precursors to a number of the chemicals that produce inflammation in the body. Unfortunately, the amount of fish oil needed to cause significant improvement in these inflammatory conditions was quite sizable and was considered too unpalatable to serve as a treatment for most people over a long period of time.

Surgery For Obesity Causing Arthritis

Several years ago, *bowel bypass surgery* was frequently done to help obese patients lose weight. Part of the small intestine where most food nutrients are absorbed was bypassed in a surgical procedure to allow food to pass through the intestinal tract untouched. The idea was that if food was not being absorbed, the patient would lose a substantial amount of weight. The part of the intestine that usually does most of the food absorption was pushed off to the side, thereby creating a dead end or "blind loop." Patients did lose weight as a result of this procedure, but one of the unexpected side effects was the development of colonies of bacteria in the bypassed bowel. In a condition called *post intestinal bypass syndrome,* particles of these bacteria would enter from the bypass into the bloodstream, causing fever, joint pain and swelling, rash, and muscle aches often so severe that the patient would have to undergo surgery to correct the surgery performed in the first place.

Needless to say, very few of these operations are performed nowadays.

Foods That Aggravate Arthritis: Are You Allergic?

For food to be nutritious, it must first cross the wall of the gastrointestinal tract into the circulation. The immune system may recognize certain foods as foreign proteins, thus provoking a response in the body. Certain diseases resulting from food or gut bacteria entering the circulation may cause significant arthritis. We have already discussed *postintestinal bypass syndrome.* With *inflammatory bowel disease,* the patient's intestinal lining becomes severely irritated, often causing diarrhea, fever, bleeding, and other serious complications. As with postintestinal bypass syndrome, inflammatory bowel disease causes the penetration of the barrier between the bloodstream and undenatured food proteins—that is, food stuffs that have not yet been broken down by the bacteria in the intestine. The bacterial protein in the gut may also gain relatively free access to the bloodstream. Excess absorption of essentially intact foodstuffs and/or bacterial protein may be the reason why many patients who suffer with *inflammatory bowel disease* have joint pain.

Diet and Rheumatoid Arthritis

Various foods have been claimed to cause or aggravate arthritis. Sodium nitrate, milk, cheese, tartrazine, wheat, corn, and beef may aggravate rheumatoid arthritis. Black walnuts have been reported to provoke both rheumatoid arthritis and another inflammatory condition known as *Behcet's disease.* One research study showed improvement in rheumatoid arthritis in two patients by eliminating from the diet red meat, fruit, dairy products, herbs, spices, additives, preservatives, and alcohol, suggesting the possibility that in at least a few cases, diet may play an important role not only in aggravating rheumatoid arthritis, but in its treatment as well.

Another study shows that milk may exacerbate preexisting rheumatoid arthritis in some patients. Milk or a placebo in the form of unmarked capsules was administered to a patient. In this double-blind study—neither the patient nor the researcher knew which capsule was which—it was discovered that in some patients the rheumatoid arthritis flared only after consuming the milk capsules.

Thus, certain foods can aggravate rheumatoid arthritis in at least some patients. In patients with such high levels of sensitivity, the best treatment seems to be avoidance.

Vitamins

As noted, a number of vitamins are necessary for the proper function of the immune system. In this section, we will consider vitamin deficiency as well as vitamin excess and see how these conditions manifest in terms of aches, pain, and fatigue. Inadequate diet is the major cause of vitamin deficiency; however, certain drugs and physical conditions may affect adversely the absorption and metabolism of vitamins in the body. For example, the alcoholic whose diet is primarily alcohol will most likely be found to be missing those vitamins not found in alcohol. But with an increased awareness of the need for vitamins and the resultant trend toward megavitamin consumption, we have also had a chance to gauge the detrimental effects of vitamin abuse. Just another case of "too much of a good thing."

Vitamins fall into two categories: water soluble and fat soluble. The first group includes vitamins Bl, B2, B3, B6, B12, and folate, while the second consists of vitamins A, D, E, and K.

Table 2 lists the major vitamins and the effects of deficiency and excess. This chart also lists the common foods in which these vitamins are found, and particular medications or conditions associated with deficiencies of any or all of these vitamins.

Look at table 2 by first examining the symptoms of deficiency. If you have any listed symptoms, check the related entry carefully. Does your diet include foods containing the vitamin? You may have a condition that affects vitamin levels or a medication that diminishes the amount of the vitamin in your body. Sometimes simply using a vitamin supplement is not sufficient to ensure that enough of the vitamin is being absorbed by the body.

Table 2 also contains the effects of vitamin excess. This can occur not only from megavitamin abuse; it may also result from consuming too much foodstuffs containing the vitamin. Vitamin supplementation or abstention (whatever the need may be) may be helpful as both a diagnostic and a treatment procedure. However, a blood test is the surest way of identifying a vitamin imbalance.

Vitamin B1 (thiamine)

Thiamine deficiency leads to *beriberi,* a disease that was fairly prevalent in East Asia in the 1800s because the factory-polished rice so basic to the diet of the region lacked the vitamin Bl. Today, beriberi is found primarily among alcohol abusers whose diet is thiamine deficient.

Beriberi involves the nervous system, resulting in burning, tingling, or numbness of the hands and/or feet *(peripheral neuropathy)*. In addition, effects on the nervous system may lead to fatigue, muscle weakness, paralysis, personality changes, depression, and decreased short- or long-term memory.

In extreme cases, thiamine deficiency may cause heart failure, palpitations, loss of appetite, and constipation. Particularly among active alcoholics, thiamine deficiency can result in severe and permanent brain dysfunction, part of which may manifest itself as a loss of contact with reality.

Excess thiamine, in those rare cases when it does occur (usually as a result of megavitamin abuse), may cause an unusual constellation of symptoms that simulate an overactive thyroid *(hyperthyroidism)*. Like hyperthyroidism, thiamine excess can cause rapid heartbeat, weakness, sweating, and poor sleep.

Vitamin B2 (riboflavin)

Riboflavin deficiency is often accompanied by other vitamin deficiencies, such as that of vitamin B3 (niacin; see below). Lack of riboflavin usually leads to skin problems, the most common of which is a cracking at the corners of the mouth called cheilosis. In addition, anyone lacking riboflavin may experience a swollen and red tongue, a sore mouth, cracked lips, a greasy scaly rash (usually on the face, but sometimes on the torso, arms, and/or legs as well) and burning itching eyes. Various medications and minerals that may influence the riboflavin levels in the individual are cited in table 2.

Vitamin B3 (niacin or nicotinic acid)

Deficiency of niacin results in *pellagra,* which is Italian for "rough skin." Pellagra produces a red rash that resembles sunburn in sun-exposed areas of the skin. Niacin deficiency can cause scaly, cracking skin *(dermatitis),* sore and swollen tongue, *diarrhea,* and *dementia* (the loss of mental faculties).

Niacin in high doses is currently used as a cholesterol-lowering agent. It is also used for treating ringing in the ears *(tinnitus)*. At such high doses, niacin can cause face-flushing, faintness, and liver damage. And because it elevates the level of uric acid in the blood, it can also cause *gout.*

Vitamin B6 (pyridoxine)

Pyridoxine deficiency may cause a greasy, scaling skin rash as well as burning, tingling, and numbness in the feet and hands *(peripheral neuropathy)*. Several common medications may lead to a relative deficiency of vitamin B6 (see table 2).

Interestingly, excess vitamin B6 has recently been associated with nerve damage, either in the form of *peripheral neuropathy,* clumsiness, headache, decreased mental ability, and seizures, as well as decreased sense of touch, temperature, position, and vibration. Arguments have been made on behalf of using pyridoxine in the treatment of *carpal tunnel syndrome, premenstrual syndrome* (PMS), and a form of anemia termed *pyridoxine-responsive sideroblastic anemia.* Some advocate using pyridoxine in the treatment of asthma and excess vomiting during pregnancy.

Interactions are of extreme importance: Patients using isoniazid, hydralazine, penicillamine, cycloserine, and oral contraceptives should have vitamin B6 supplements. In contrast, patients with *Parkinson's disease* who take levodopa should not be given vitamin B6 because this vitamin decreases the effectiveness of the medication.

Vitamin B12 (cyanocobalamin)

Vitamin B12 has been aptly nicknamed the "energy vitamin." Deficiency of this vitamin is fairly common. As described in the chapter on fatigue, vitamin B12, even when present in sufficient quantities in the diet, may not be adequately absorbed because of a lack of a protein called *intrinsic factor,* which parietal cells produce in the stomach lining. Vitamin B12, in association with sufficient intrinsic factor and adequate stomach acid, is then absorbed in the last part of the small intestine. A breakdown at any point in this mechanism may lead to a lack of B12 in the blood.

One of the manifestations of vitamin B12 deficiency is a decreased red blood cell count termed *pernicious anemia.* Prolonged B12 deficiency may result in a decrease of the white blood cell count as well as platelets in the blood. The individual may feel burning, tingling, and numbness of the hands and feet *(peripheral neuropathy).*

It is now believed that vitamin B12 deficiency is more common than previously thought, especially among the elderly whose stomachs produce less acid. In some cases, this has led to an intellectual-mental impairment that has been misdiagnosed as *Alzheimer's disease.* Proper diagnosis in vitamin B12 deficiency is urgent, because nerve and brain damage may become permanent if not treated early.

It has been shown that elevation of certain blood proteins (methylmalonic acid and homocysteine) is a more sensitive test for vitamin B12 deficiency than blood vitamin B12 levels. These tests may lead to earlier detection of vitamin B12 deficiency.

Tragically, patients with vitamin B12 deficiency given high-dose folic acid may experience improvement in their low blood counts and yet continue to suffer profound nerve and brain damage. To prevent such masking of B12 deficiency, high-dose folic acid is only available by prescription.

Injections of vitamin B12 circumvent the absorption problem and provide easy, effective treatment.

Vitamin B12 has been controversially used as a health tonic and a treatment for *multiple sclerosis* and *trigeminal neuralgia.* No side effects from excess use have been described thus far.

Vitamin C (ascorbic acid)

There are two things that humans, monkeys, and guinea pigs have in common: All three species lack the ability to produce vitamin C within the body, and all three thus may experience vitamin C deficiency.

Vitamin C deficiency or scurvy has been known since the Crusades. British sailors became known as "limeys" when lime juice was added to their diet in the late 18th century as a preventative against scurvy. Before then, British sailors deprived of the usual sources of vitamin C (citrus fruits, tomatoes) succumbed to weakness, fatigue, and anemia as well as excess bleeding and bruising.

Vitamin C in large doses has been touted as a cure or a preventative for everything from the common cold to cancer. Unfortunately, studies up to this point have not clearly demonstrated the effective of megadose vitamin C for these purposes. While vitamin C has been used successfully in the treatment of two rare disorders, *Ehlers-Danlos syndrome* (a disorder of the body's connective tissue) and *Chediak-Higashi syndrome* (a disorder affecting white blood cell function), the only effects of megadose vitamin C discovered so far are an increase in the incidence of kidney stones and an increase in the absorption of iron. Vitamin C may also decrease copper levels and decrease the effectiveness of tricylic antidepressants. Chewable vitamin C may erode dental enamel.

It is important to note that stopping megadose vitamin C may cause a rebound deficiency state, resulting in scurvy. This can affect newborn babies whose mothers took excessive vitamin C during pregnancy. There have also been suggestions that excess vitamin C may increase cholesterol levels and deactivate vitamin B12.

Folic Acid (folate)

Folic acid, like vitamin B12 is absorbed in the small bowel. Therefore, small bowel disease will affect folic acid absorption as well. Folic acid deficiency may cause *anemia* (decreased red blood cell count), burning tongue, and fatigue. Folic acid is present in many foods; however, prolonged cooking may destroy much of this vitamin.

Vitamin A

Vitamin A is one of the four fat-soluble vitamins that require bile (produced in the liver) to be absorbed properly in the intestine. The other fat-soluble vitamins are K, D, and E. All these vitamins may become deficient if a diseased liver does not produce enough bile. However, certain medications used to lower cholesterol (colestipol, for example, and cholestyramine) may bind up the bile; therefore, a side effect may be poor absorption of either fats or fat-soluble vitamins. Likewise, if the bowel is damaged and does not absorb the fat or if the pancreas fails to produce the fat-emulsifying enzyme lipase, vitamin deficiency may occur even when adequate amounts of vitamins A, D, E, and K are present in the diet.

Vitamin A deficiency is still common in undeveloped countries because of poor diet. Decreased vision, especially at night, dry eyes, blindness, roughened skin, and bone pain are effects of this deficiency.

Excess vitamin A may occur with megavitamin A abuse, excessive fish oil intake, using vitamin A with retinoids (acne medication), and by using vitamin A with oral contraceptives. An increase of vitamin A levels in the body may cause fatigue, dry and coarse skin, muscle aches, increased pressure in the brain, liver disease, and bone pain due to excessive bony growth.

Given the complications of vitamin A abuse over an extended period of time, it is not surprising that a sudden and massive overdose of vitamin A is extremely dangerous. There are reports of a team of Arctic explorers who killed a polar bear and ate its liver, an especially rich source of vitamin A. They suffered severe swelling in the brain, peeling of the skin, and ultimately, a truly horrible death.

Vitamin A derivatives are used successfully to treat several skin diseases, most notably *acne* and *psoriasis*. It is also used to promote wound healing.

Vitamin K

Vitamin K is an agent involved in the formation of several important proteins of blood clotting. In humans and most animals, bacteria in the intestine produce vitamin K. However, antibiotics may destroy these bacteria, thus causing a vitamin K deficiency. And as with vitamin A, bile dysfunction causing the impediment of fat absorption can also affect levels of vitamin K. Deficiency of vitamin K results in excessive bruising and bleeding.

Vitamin K is so effective in its association with blood clotting that medications designed to thin the blood when blood clots may be problematic or even fatal are directed against it. Such is the case of warfarin, a drug which competes with vitamin K in the liver, thereby affecting the production of certain clotting factors.

Warfarin has proven so effective in this capacity that it has become the most popular rat poison in the world. Consequently, in human treatment, the medication must be used with great caution.

Vitamin E

Vitamin E, another fat-soluble vitamin whose absorption depends on the liver, bile, pancreas, and intestine, has come to be known as the "fertility vitamin" because it is essential in both males and females for reproduction among rats and other mammals. However, this has never been shown to be true in humans. Vitamin E deficiency in humans manifests as muscle weakness and decreased red blood cell count. Vitamin E excess may result in fatigue, headache, and muscle weakness. Vitamin E has been used successfully to treat *muscle, cramps* and the painful breasts of *fibrocystic breast disease.*

Vitamin D

Vitamin D, the last of the fat-soluble vitamins, is produced in sun-exposed skin and is activated in the liver and the kidney. Lack of adequate sunlight or a poorly functioning liver or kidney may decrease the effectiveness of vitamin D. In addition, phenytoin and barbiturates may decrease the liver metabolism of vitamin D, which in turn will result in a lessening of the effectiveness of vitamin D present in the body. Vitamin D is involved closely in calcium metabolism. Deficiency of vitamin

D in children causes *rickets,* a condition in which the bones have too little calcium. This leaves the bones soft, causing the legs to bend into a bowlegged deformity. *Adult rickets* or *osteomalacia* results from vitamin D deficiency in adults after the bones have normally formed. Lacking adequate calcium, the bones fracture easily and cause pain. The patient may also have difficulty rising from a chair or climbing stairs.

Excess vitamin D may result in increased blood calcium levels which may in turn cause excessive urination as well as kidney stones. The bones may become weak and brittle as excess vitamin D tends to cause increased resorption of calcium directly from the bones.

Vitamin D is used as a medication to treat vitamin D deficiency and to increase blood calcium levels where circumstances call for it.

Minerals

As with vitamins, minerals also figure in our needs for a balanced diet. And as with vitamins, certain medications, the lack of key foods, or other special circumstances may lead to mineral deficiency. Not all of the known minerals are covered in this section—only those that in deficient or excessive quantities produce weakness, fatigue, or discomfort. As in the section on vitamins, we have included a table describing the possible effects of having too few or too many minerals. With this table, you may correlate your physical symptoms, any medications you may be using and a variety of special conditions with the levels of minerals in your body. The medications are listed in the generic form. Blood levels of minerals may be determined by laboratory testing. As you will see, significant problems can occur with deficient or excessive states of minerals in the body.

Table 2
Vitamin Deficiency and Excess States

Vitamin	Effects Of Deficiency	Effects of Excess	Foods Containing the Vitamin	Medications/ Conditions That Decrease Body Levels or Effects of the Vitamin
B1 thiamine	burning, ting-ling, numbness of hand and/or feet (peripheral neuropathy), decreased red blood cells count (anemia), fatigue, head-ache, weak-ness, decreased mental ability, weakened heart muscle, constipation	headache, weakness difficulty sleeping, rapid heart rate, trembling	beef, pork, liver, whole grains, enriched cereal, peas, beans, nuts	antacids, raw fish, seafood, dialysis, alcohol abuse, poor diet, polished rice diet
B2 riboflavin	decreased red blood cell count (anemia), sore mouth, swollen/ red tongue, cracked lips/corners of mouth, burning/ itching eyes, greasy/ scaly skin rash.	burning, numbness, tingling; other unusual sensations.	milk, milk products, fruits, vegetables, meats, liver, grains.	ascorbic acid (vitamin c), iron, erythromycin, streptomycin, doxorubicin, copper, imipramine, chloropromazine zinc, saccharin, oral contraceptives, tryptophan, alcohol abuse, low thyroid (hypothyroid), chronic diarrhea, large skin burns

Vitamin	Effects Of Deficiency	Effects of Excess	Foods Containing the Vitamin	Medications/ Conditions That Decrease Body Levels or Effects of the Vitamin
B3 niacin	sore mouth/ tongue, abdominal discomfort, burning, tingling, numbness (nerve inflammation), weakness, "spinning" dizziness (vertigo), diarrhea, decreased mental ability, convulsions, red rash in sun-exposed areas.	heart rhythm problems, increased uric acid (may cause gout), face flushing, dry, itchy skin, abdominal pain, liver damage, increased skin pigment, faintness	meats, milk, eggs, peanuts, enriched grains.	6 mercaptopurine, isoniazid, oral contraceptives, deficiency of vitamin B6, leucine, alcohol abuse, excess corn in the diet, chronic diarrhea
B6 pyri-doxine	burning, tingling, numbness of hands and/or feet (peripheral neuropathy), decreased red blood cell count (anemia), dizziness, weakness, diarrhea, swollen/red tongue, cracked lips/ corner of mouth, kidney stones, greasy/ scaly skin rash	burning, tingling, numbness of hands and/or feet (peripheral neuropathy), headache, fatigue, clum-siness, de-creased mental ability, decreas-ed sense of touch tempera-ture/ position, vibration/numb-ness around the mouth, seizures, ulcers	liver, kidney meat, wheat, nuts, beans, fruits, grains, vegetables	isoniazid, hydralazine, penicillamine, cycloserine, oral contraceptives, levodopa, alcohol abuse, excess protein intake

Vitamin	Effects Of Deficiency	Effects of Excess	Foods Containing the Vitamin	Medications/ Conditions That Decrease Body Levels or Effects of the Vitamin
B12 cyano- cobalami n	burning, tingling, numbness of hands and/or feet (peripheral neuropathy), sore mouth/ tongue, decreased red blood cell county (anemia), decreased sense of touch/position/tas te/ smell/visual acuity, decreased mental ability, lemon tint to skin		meat, liver, fish, eggs, milk, cheese	cimetidine, colchicine, ranitidine, pernicious anemia, stomach removal (partial or complete) ileitis or other intestinal diseases, surgery that produces a "dead-end" or blind loop of small intestine, fish tapeworm, chronic disease of the pancreas, strict vegetarian diet
Folate folic acid	decreased red blood cell count (anemia), burning tongue, fatigue	decreased zinc level	spinach, lettuce, asparagus, broccoli, liver, kidneys, yeast, mushrooms	aluminum antacids, oral contraceptives, phenobarbital, phenytoin, methotrexate, sulfasalazine, trimethoprim, cholestyromine, colestipol, triamterene, alcohol abuse, malabsorption (intestinal disease), lack of vegetables in diet, dialysis, excessive cooking of food

213

Vitamin	Effects Of Deficiency	Effects of Excess	Foods Containing the Vitamin	Medications/ Conditions That Decrease Body Levels or Effects of the Vitamin
C	fatigue, weakness, pain in joints/bones, bleeding into joints, bleeding/ swollen/sore gums, burning, tingling, numbness (nerve damage), excess bruising, decreased red blood cell count (anemia), poor wound healing	kidney stones, poor sleep, fatigue, headache, diarrhea, hot flashes, stomach upset	citrus (grapefruits, oranges, lemons, lime), asparagus, turnip greens, chili peppers, tomatoes, cabbage, potatoes, strawberries	alcohol abuse, oral contraceptives, lack of proper food in diet, dialysis, excess cooked food in diet (vitamin C is heat sensitive)
A	painful bones, headache, decreased vision (especially at night), dry eyes, loss of sense of taste, rough skin, kidney stones	dry, itchy, coarse skin, sore mouth, headache, painful bones/ joints, fatigue, increased blood calcium levels, liver damage, yellow-orange skin, decreased mental ability, increased pressure in the brain	carrots, sweet potatoes, leafy green vegetables, yams, yellow corn, yellow squash, apricots, palm oils, peaches, fish liver oils, kidney, eggs, milk	cholestyramine, colestipol, neomycin, colchicine, mineral oil, clofibrate, alcohol abuse, poor diet, chronic laxative use (especially mineral oil), zinc deficiency, poor absorption of fats, liver disease, diseases of the intestine, cystic fibrosis

Vitamin	Effects Of Deficiency	Effects of Excess	Foods Containing the Vitamin	Medications/ Conditions That Decrease Body Levels or Effects of the Vitamin
K	bleeding easy bruising		vegetables (especially turnip greens, broccoli, brussels sprouts, spinach, lettuce), moderate amounts present in: egg yolk, liver, bacon, cheese, butter, coffee, green tea	warfarin, mineral oil, laxatives, tetracycline, colestipol, cholestyramine resin, phenytoin, phenobarbital, primidone, poor absorption of fats, liver disease
E	muscle weakness, decreased sense of vibration /position, weak eye muscles, decreased red blood cell count (anemia)	fatigue, diarrhea, muscle weakness, headache, dizziness, faintness	soybean, corn, cottonseed, wheat germ, safflower oils, vegetable oils, milk, eggs, cereals, leafy vegetables, meat, fish	mineral oil, cholestyramine, colestipol, severe malabsorption, poor absorption of fats, cystic fibrosis, celiac disease, Crohn's disease
D	poor calcium absorption, in adults causes osteomalacia (defective bone mineralization); bone pain, muscle weakness, (difficulty arising from chair or climbing stairs), in children causes rickets (malformed bones)	fatigue, weakness, headaches, abdominal cramps, fragile bones/bone pain, kidney stones, increased calcium levels, excess urination	dairy products, fish oils	phenytoin, mineral oil, barbiturates, isoniazid, phenolphthalein, colestipol, cholestyramine, aluminum antacids, poor absorption of fats, lack of sunlight, severe, kidney or liver disease

Sodium

Sodium plays a number of vital roles in the body. It balances the body's water and acidity, it affects muscle action, it helps the body absorb energy-giving glucose in the intestine, and it plays a role in the maintenance of blood pressure.

Thus, it is very much in the body's interest to maintain the sodium concentration in the blood. However, certain medications (see table 2) and diseases *(tuberculosis, lung cancer, brain tumors)* may disrupt these mechanisms and cause a decrease in sodium concentration in the blood. Similarly, *diarrhea* and *sweating* will deplete the body of sodium.

Other causes of low sodium include low thyroid hormone (hypothyroid) and low output of cortisol (the body's natural "cortisone") from the adrenal gland. This is called *Addison's disease.*

Interestingly, both too little and too much sodium concentration has similar effects: sleepiness, fatigue, seizures, even coma. Low sodium is a common cause of *muscle cramps.*

While many experts advocate a low sodium diet to treat high blood pressure, the body's ability to conserve sodium is so good that low blood sodium does not usually occur on such diets.

Aside from recognizing that cramps, seizures, and sleepiness may be caused by abnormalities in sodium balance, an early search for the cause of such problems is important, since they can often be manifestations of significant medical problems.

Potassium

Potassium is a mineral that serves a number of vital purposes. Like sodium, for example, it plays a role in the preservation of the water balance and blood pressure and contributes to muscle function. Potassium is also involved in metabolic reactions— regulating the synthesis and storage of glucose, for example.

The critical role of potassium is reflected in the very tight range demanded of the mineral in the blood. Potassium deficiency or excess may cause a decrease in body muscle tone, weakness, and abnormal heart rhythm. Low potassium may cause fatigue, weakening of the heart muscle, heart failure, and deterioration in kidney function. Numerous medications may affect potassium levels (see table 3). Among causes of potassium deficiency are prolonged vomiting or diarrhea, low potassium in the diet, or a superabundant output of cortisol from the adrenal gland (otherwise known as *Cushing's disease* or *syndrome).* Licorice and chewing tobacco have both been found to contain a chemical that decreases the body's potassium.

Causes of increased potassium levels include excessive intake (either orally or by injection), kidney failure, and those medications that inhibit the normal excretion of potassium by the kidney.

As with sodium abnormalities, you should be examined properly for the underlying cause of either high or low potassium. Your life may depend on it.

Fluoride

Fluoride is a mineral which in small quantities has been proven to prevent tooth decay. Its use at higher doses for the treatment of thin bones *(osteoporosis)* is still experimental. Fluoride may increase the total amount of bone, but the newly formed bone is not as strong as normal bone. Such high doses of fluoride as the experimental treatment requires may cause mottling of the teeth, stomach ulcers, bone breakage, and inflammation of the palms, soles, and joints.

Zinc

Zinc is a mineral currently undergoing a great deal of scrutiny as a possible treatment for various ailments. For example, it is used on the skin to treat such conditions as dandruff and acne. It is also used for treating *acrodermatitis enteropathica,* a rare rash that results from a genetic defect in the absorption of zinc. Some hint as to its possible restorative powers are indicated by the wide variety of symptoms that become apparent in the course of zinc deficiency. Decreased zinc

217

levels lead to poor wound healing, *diarrhea,* decreased mental ability, decreased senses of taste and smell, scaly rashes, and fatigue. Decreased zinc may be caused by poor dietary intake, poor absorption in the intestine, and excessive sweating. Penicillamine, a drug used for the treatment of rheumatoid arthritis, may bind up zinc, thereby decreasing levels.

Excess zinc may occur from over ingestion as well as from occupational exposure (industrial fumes, for example). Zinc excess may result in fatigue and *anemia* (decreased red blood cell count).

Copper

Copper deficiency rarely occurs in humans. Penicillamine, excess vitamin C, excess zinc, and bowel diseases are causes of decreased copper. Low levels of copper in the body may lead to a decrease in red blood cell count *(anemia)* and a decreased sensation of taste and smell.

Excess copper occurs in *Wilson's disease,* a congenital condition in which the body accumulates abnormal amounts of copper. The copper may be concentrated in the liver or in the nervous system, causing liver disease, restricted coordination, and/or decreased mental ability. Muscle aches and *anemia* may also occur with excess copper in the body. Abnormal kidney function may also occur.

Copper has been reported to help arthritis, particularly in the use of bracelets worn on the forearm; however, such claims have never been scientifically substantiated.

Selenium

Selenium is a minor mineral whose deficiency has been associated with muscle aching and a weakening of the heart. Very large doses of selenium may cause a metallic taste in the mouth, a bronze color to the skin, brittle nails and hair, as well as fatigue.

Magnesium

Magnesium is a mineral whose importance to the body is only now coming to be appreciated. It is involved in the general metabolism of the body, most notably in catalyzing reactions that produce energy, producing body compounds, as well as in the transportation and absorption of nutrients. It plays a role in protein synthesis, muscle action, and thyroid and parathyroid hormone secretion.

Magnesium deficiency may occur after prolonged diarrhea or vomiting, lack of magnesium in the diet, alcohol abuse, and use of certain medications, notably water pills. Deficiency results in fatigue, weakness, decreased mental capabilities, burning, numbness, tingling, lowered calcium levels, and convulsions.

Along with its uses as a laxative and an antacid, magnesium is used to treat an emergency condition during pregnancy called *eclampsia*. This condition produces severely high blood pressure that can endanger both mother and fetus.

Excess magnesium levels may occur through the overuse of certain antacids and laxatives. Lithium may also provoke excessive magnesium. Another possible cause of increased magnesium is kidney disease. Excess magnesium may cause fatigue, weakness, decreased blood pressure, decreased heart rate, and even total heart stoppage in extreme circumstances.

Phosphate

Phosphate is important for bone and tooth formation, energy metabolism, and maintenance of the body's acid/base balance. Body stores of phosphate may be depleted by alcohol abuse, antacids that bind phosphates, and kidney dialysis. The resultant deficiency can produce weakness, pain in the bones, red blood cell destruction, burning, tingling, numbness, and convulsions.

The most common cause of iron loss is bleeding, either menstrual or via the intestinal tract (for example, ulcers, stomach inflammation or colon growths called *polyps).* Iron absorption depends on adequate acid levels in the stomach; thus, the iron level will be affected by the use of antacids or by any surgery that removes part or all of the stomach. Certain medications may also deplete iron levels (see Table 3), resulting in *anemia,* fatigue, inflamed tongue, and cracked corners of the mouth. It may also result in *pica,* the craving of nonfood material, including ice, dirt, and clay.

Excessive iron may occur with the over ingestion of iron, numerous blood transfusions, and a genetic disease called *hemochromatosis.* In *hemochromatosis,* the excess iron is absorbed into various organs: in the pancreas, it produces *diabetes;* in the liver, it destroys tissue and on occasion can cause cancer. The skin may turn a bronze color, and the joints may become loaded with iron, causing stiffness and swelling, particularly in the knuckles of the hands. Excess iron may produce heart failure and rhythm abnormalities. Undetected and untreated, hemochromatosis can lead to significant destructive change, but if detected early, the effects are reversible.

Iodine (iodide)

Iodine is reduced to iodide in the intestinal tract before it is absorbed. Once inside the body, iodide is absorbed by the thyroid gland, located in the neck. This gland produces thyroid hormone which is closely involved with the body metabolism. When the body lacks iodide, the thyroid gland may produce too little hormone, leading to a low thyroid condition. The individual may experience an increased sensitivity to cold, muscle weakness, fatigue, poor memory, slowed heart rate, dry skin, and sluggish speech. The thyroid gland may enlarge in such cases, causing what is called a *goiter.* In the past, such deficiencies were more apt to occur in land-locked regions such as Switzerland where there is less access to seafood. With the introduction of iodinated table salt, iodide deficiency has become far less common.

Iodide excess may occur from taking expectorants used to make respiratory secretions more liquid. Iodide may cause acne as well as swelling and/or discomfort of the salivary glands, particularly in the parotid gland. Located in front of each ear, the parotid is the chief source of saliva. Excess iodide may paradoxically cause the thyroid gland to swell, thereby leading to a decrease in thyroid hormone.

Iodine may cause allergic reactions, especially when administered in the form of contrast agents for use in X-ray studies. It can slow down an overactive thyroid gland *(hyperthyroidism)* when used in the radioactive form. The radioactive form concentrates in the thyroid gland where it destroys the overactive thyroid gland permanently.

Iodide may also be used to treat a fungus condition called sporotrichosis.

Calcium

Calcium makes up most of our bones and also has important functions in both nerve and muscle tissue. Vitamin D and the hormone produced by the parathyroid gland in the neck (parathormone) are two keys to the body's calcium metabolism. These work so well that even with a diet deficient in calcium, the blood calcium levels are usually held at a normal level by drawing off calcium from the bones, the chief reservoir of calcium in the body. Consequently, blood calcium levels do not accurately reflect the total body calcium stores.

Lower blood levels of calcium may result from a lack of both calcium and vitamin D, problems with the parathyroid gland, advanced kidney disease, or a lack of stomach acid. Stomach acid enhances calcium absorption, so calcium levels may be affected by the use of certain medications, for example, to treat ulcers. Blood transfusions which contain the chemical citrate may lower the blood calcium level because citrate binds up calcium. Magnesium deficiency may cause low calcium because magnesium is needed for normal parathyroid hormone secretion.

Low blood calcium levels may lead to a number of problems. The bones may weaken and become susceptible to breaking. You may feel numbness and tingling in the fingertips and around the mouth. Low calcium may also lead to tetany, a state of severe muscle contraction. Low calcium can also cause cataracts, convulsions, muscle cramps, and increased pressure in the brain.

Blood calcium levels may be increased with the ingestion of excess vitamin D or calcium. Excess calcium ingestion may occur in patients who have ulcers and take large amounts of calcium-laden antacids. Thiazide diuretics (a water pill) may tend to increase blood calcium levels by decreasing the kidney excretion of calcium. Sarcoidosis, a disease usually affecting the lungs as well as other organs, may also be associated with increased calcium levels. Excess production of parathyroid hormone *(hyperparathyroidism)* may cause increased calcium levels. Cancer (particularly of the lung) may produce chemicals that increase blood calcium levels. Direct tumor invasion of the bone such as with breast cancer may also increase blood calcium levels.

Elevated blood calcium levels are capable of rendering serious damage. Severe fatigue, weakness of the muscles, poor mental functioning, and even coma may result. Kidney stones as well as kidney deterioration may occur. The pancreas may become inflamed *(pancreatitis) a*nd severe constipation may also result from excessive blood calcium levels.

Table 3
Mineral Deficiency and Excess

Mineral	Effects of Deficiency	Effects of Excess	Foods Containing the Vitamin	Medications/ Conditions That Decrease Body Levels or Effects of the Mineral
Sodium	weakness, fatigue, sleepiness, muscle cramps	fatigue, sleepiness, confusion, convulsions	table salt milk, meat, eggs, baking soda, baking powder, beets, spinach, celery	diuretics (water pills), chlorpropamide, tolbutamide, vincristine, carbamazepine, amitriptyline, theophyline, aminoglycoside antibiotics, excess diarrhea, excess sweating, low thyroid (hypothyroidism) low adrenal gland hormone (Addison's disease), tuberculosis, pneumonia, lung tumors, brain tumor, bleeding within the brain, porphyria
Potassium	weakness, fatigue, poor muscle tone, poor kidney function, weakening of heart muscle, abnormal heart rhythm	poor muscle tone, abnormal heart rhythm	whole grains, meat, legumes, fruits, vegetables	diuretics (water pills), carbenicillin, cortisone, poor diet, aminoglycoside antibiotics, phenophthalein, capreomycin, bisacodyl, amphotericin B, excess vomiting, diarrhea, low magnesium level, malnutrition, cystic fibrosis, excess adrenal gland hormones (Cushing's disease), excess licorice ingestion, excess use of chewing tobacco

Mineral	Effects of Deficiency	Effects of Excess	Foods Containing the Vitamin	Medications/ Conditions That Decrease Body Levels or Effects of the Mineral
Fluoride		inflammation of palms and soles, stomach ulcers, spontaneous bone breaks, joint inflammation, decreased red blood cell count (anemia)	fluorinated water, fish, fish products, tea	
Zinc	fatigue, decreased sense of taste/smell, poor wound healing, scaly thickened skin, diarrhea, decreased mental ability	decreased red blood cell count (anemia), fatigue	liver, seafood (especially oysters), eggs, milk, whole grains	penicillamine, alcohol abuse, liver cirrhosis, poor bowel absorption, inflammatory bowel disease (Crohn's ulcerative colitis), kidney disease, psoriasis, pancreas disease, excess sweating
Copper	decreased red blood cell count (anemia), decreased sensation of taste, loss of protein in urine	muscle aches, red blood cell destruction, liver disease, poor coordination, decreased mental ability, abnormal kidney function	liver, meats, seafood, whole grains, legumes, nuts, cocoa, raisins, food cooked in cooper utensils	excess vitamin C, excess zinc, penicillamine, cystic fibrosis, poor bowel absorption

Mineral	Effects of Deficiency	Effects of Excess	Foods Containing the Vitamin	Medications/ Conditions That Decrease Body Levels or Effects of the Mineral
Selenium	muscle aches, weakening of the heart muscle	fatigue, skin rash/bronze color to skin, brittle nails/hair, sore throat, metallic taste	seafoods, meats, whole grains, kidney, chicken, mushrooms, egg yolks, radishes	
Magnesium	fatigue, weakness, decreased mental ability, heart rhythm abnormalities, constipation, burning, numbness, tingling, other unusual sensations, convulsions, decreased calcium levels	fatigue, weakness, decreased blood pressure, decreased heart rate	green vegetables, milk, meat, fish, nuts, whole grains	cisplatinum, aminoglycoside, antibiotics, diuretic (water pills), excess vomiting, diarrhea, alcohol abuse, pancreas inflammation, starvation, poorly controlled diabetes
Phosphate	weakness, red blood cell destruction, bone pain, burning, numbness, tingling, other unusual sensations, convulsions.		milk, cheese, meat, egg yolk, whole grains	antacids that bind phosphate, alcohol abuse, dialysis, poorly controlled diabetes, excess parathyroid hormone

Mineral	Effects of Deficiency	Effects of Excess	Foods Containing the Vitamin	Medications/ Conditions That Decrease Body Levels or Effects of the Mineral
Iron	decreased red blood cell count (anemia), fatigue, inflamed tongue, cracks at mouth corners, pica (unnatural cravings, especially for ice, dirt, clay)	joint pain, diabetes, liver disease, bronze skin, constipation, weakened heart muscle, heart rhythm problems	liver, meats, egg yolks, whole grains, nuts, enriched bread and cereal, legumes	phosphase, neo-mycin, dactino-mycin, antacids with carbonates, choles-tyramine, penicil-lamine, aspirin, nonsteroidal anti-inflammatory drugs, lack of stomach acid, partial or complete stomach removal, excess bleeding (from the intestines, stomach, menstrual periods, for example), excess tea (phytate) ingestion,
Iodine	enlarged thy-roid (goiter), hypothyroidism, increased sen-sitivity to cold, muscle weak-ness, fatigue, poor memory, slow pulse, dry skin, slow speech	acne, salivary gland enlargement/ pain	iodinized salt, seafood	iodine deficient diet
Calcium	numbness/ tingling around mouth and fingertips, weak and thinned bones, cata-racts, conv-ulsions, in-creased pres-sure in the brain, muscle cramps, tetany	severe fatigue weakness, decreased mental ability, kidney stones, const-ipation, ex-cess urina-tion, pancreas inflammation, decreased liver function	milk, cheese, green leafy vegetables whole grains.	dactinomycin, lack of stomach acid, magnesium defic-iency, blood trans-fusions with citrated blood, vitamin D deficiency combined with calcium deficient diet, dis-ease or surgical removal of para-thryroid gland

Most of us know that medications have potential side-effects. Most of these have been identified in lab and clinical trials and are included in the *Physician's Desk Reference;* however, even the PDR cannot anticipate unusual responses to medications, particularly when various medications are being taken simultaneously. It is impossible to chart all possible permutations of medication, combined dosages, and physical effects.

Due to the extremely large number of available drugs and potential interactions we recommend that the reader apply for a free subscription to Epocrates[R]. This is downloadable software that will describe drug side effects – common and severe. It will also enable you to put your medications into the interaction tool to see if your medications may be causing problems with each other. As physicians, we find this resource to be indispensable.

For certain drug side-effects, there may be more information available elsewhere in this book. For example, if a drug is listed as potentially causing low sodium, information regarding the effects of decreased blood sodium will be found in chapter 10, "Vitamins, Minerals, Diet, and Nutrition." Likewise, if a drug has the potential for causing muscle inflammation, further information on that condition may be found in chapter 6, "Muscle Pain and Weakness." Check the index to see if the condition cited here is referred to elsewhere.

Whatever you do, act at least with the advice of your physician. If you feel that your medications are causing side-effects you cannot tolerate, consult your physician immediately; do not take it upon yourself to stop treatment. Other medications are generally available for treatment, but please do not hazard stopping your treatment all together.

Choosing a doctor is one of the most important decisions you ever have to make, yet most people are ill prepared to make that decision in an intelligent and informed manner. Circumstances often work against the patient: In seeking quick relief from suffering, you may choose a doctor simply on the basis of which one is available soonest. Sadly, it is difficult to get a sense of the quality of a doctor's care giving until you are actually in the office.

Another problem working against the patient is the way in which many private medical insurance programs provide the subscriber access only to a limited number of participating physicians. When you sign on, you are often forced to sign up with a primary-care physician without the benefit of interviewing the doctor beforehand. Subsequent efforts to change primary-care physicians may be hampered by bureaucratic restrictions placed by the contract provider.

Whatever prompts your decision to choose a doctor, the purpose is, if you are ill, to feel better. Moreover, once you are well, you still want a doctor who will help you maintain your sense of being well. For the purpose of this book, we are assuming that you are seeking a doctor for treatment. As we have noted, correct treatment can only follow correct diagnosis; therefore, the physician you choose should be the one most capable of getting to the bottom of your problem.

An ailing person has two possible avenues to pursue in the search for a good physician. On the one hand, you can go to a family physician to discuss the situation. After an examination and evaluation of your situation, the family physician may either address the condition or recommend you to a specialist.

On the other hand, you may choose to go directly to a specialist. The question then becomes which type of specialist you should visit. If the problem is occurring in a *single joint*—for example, the shoulder—it would be appropriate to see an orthopedic doctor or a rheumatologist. *If more than one joint is affected or if several muscle areas ache,* the rheumatologist might be a better choice, as his is a specialty that concentrates on diseases affecting multiple joints, muscles, and soft tissues. After you have considered your situation carefully and have determined that your problem revolves around *weakness and fatigue,* a family practitioner or an internist might provide the best initial evaluation of your condition.

Finally, if the nature of your discomfort is associated with *burning, tingling, numbness,* or *dizziness,* a neurologist would be the best doctor to start with.

These are, of course, generalizations, and many specialists and family physicians treat the same medical conditions.

What About the Doctor?

Okay, you've now gotten a group of referrals. How do you select one doctor out of several, any one of whom could treat your condition?

An obvious, important, but not entirely necessary consideration is whether he or she has board certification. Similarly, where did the physician do his or her training? Though important, these qualifications should not be the only criteria upon which to base your selection. Many physicians who have not trained at the best medical schools or who have not received board certification in any particular realm of specialization can still be excellent diagnosticians.

For example, one issue to bear in mind is the age of the physician and the length of time he or she has been out of training. Some physicians are better than others at keeping abreast of the latest medical research in their areas, though they received their formal medical education quite some time ago. Others find that as their practices develop, they begin to engage in areas of expertise that were not part of their original training. This is especially true for physicians who have become involved with a particular clientele.

229

In the end, the physician you are really seeking is the one who is experienced in treating patients with aches and pains. You should look for a physician who will talk to you and look you in the eye as he or she is talking. You should also seek out a physician who will listen to you and consider what you know and feel in terms of the overall diagnostic and treatment plan.

Physician Personality Traits

Certain character traits make for better doctors. Much of good diagnosis comes from a desire to get to the bottom of things. There are, unfortunately, not a few physicians who will arrive at a diagnosis and stop looking at the full extent of the symptoms. Having made their minds up as to what is wrong with the patient, they are not going to do any further investigation. All of this is fine when they are right—say, eighty-five percent of the time—but you might want a different doctor if you fall within the other fifteen.

If you don't know what's wrong with you—or even if you do—the physician capable of coming to grips with the changing meaning of arthritis is one who is willing to take into account all the possible factors of your illness. Such a physician will not arrive at a diagnosis prematurely; rather, he or she will become a driving force behind finding the right diagnosis and treatment for you.

What this means is that the physician must be willing to say, "I don't know." Where those words might seem shameful for some, for others it makes the difficult diagnostic problem a challenge and not a burden to avoid.

Finally, there is the old ideal of the doctor as the omniscient, personable, nice person who will spend all kinds of time with a single patient. While these traits are important—the patient does, after all, want to be able to have confidence in his or her physician— the reality of modern medical practice makes this almost impossible. In a world where doctors are faced with soaring insurance rates and shrinking third-party payments, most physicians must see a large number of patients daily to cover their increasing overhead.

Trust: The Core of Doctor-Patient Relations

The issue is trust. The old vision of the doctor carried with it the notion that the patient trusted the doctor implicitly, immediately, simply because he or she was a doctor. The ways of modern medicine have changed that forever, and the doctor-patient relationship has had to change with them.

The good doctor-patient relationship is a two-way street. Physicians and their staff do not look upon angry, rude patients fondly. The "squeaky wheel" may get the grease but often risks getting the boot. Be persistent, by all means—do whatever you have to to get well—but also be polite. As you enter into a relationship with your doctor, both of you will get the most out of a sense of cooperation.

And perhaps the most difficult thing of all is being patient. Some diagnoses are not that easy to make—for example, with over 100 different causes for arthritis, the doctor needs time as well as information to help you. Similarly, certain treatments require a long time to take effect. The notion of waiting may be difficult when you endure pain, but bear in mind that poor treatment can be worse than no treatment at all.

Medical treatment is part science, part art. Given the complexity of the human body, technique in diagnosis stems as much from intuition as it does from clear observation and lab work. Consequently, the answers you sometimes get from your doctor are not as well defined as you would like them to be. In a good therapeutic relationship, however, the answer will become sharper when you and the doctor work together.

Where Do You Start?

There is no perfect place to begin your search. Your general physician, the internet, or a local hospital physician finder service— any one of these may be fruitful. Often, the best place to start is a friend's recommendation. You now have some idea of the right questions to ask—was the diagnosis correct? Did the treatment work? Was the physician sympathetic or completely uninterested? The sooner you put them to use, the sooner you will find yourself the right doctor.

Remember Your Original Goal

Your purpose is to find the best possible treatment for your condition. As we have said, the first step in getting that treatment is being properly diagnosed. You will want a careful and thorough examination, after which you will have to gauge how well the doctor's conclusion jibes with your own sense of the problem.

If either you or your physician is less than satisfied with the diagnosis, the treatment, or the outcome of the treatment, both of you must consider the possibility of further evaluation by another doctor—be it a specialist or a researcher at a university medical center.

Somewhere along the line, most patients find that elusive answer. To reach that point sooner, bring all the knowledge you can muster to bear on the problem of making the wise choice in selecting your doctor. The results may be sometimes frustrating at first, but if you persist and seek all advice where possible, the selection of the right doctor will be the most important first step in the treatment of your ailment.

Aches and pain, particularly those due to arthritis, may be associated with many other diseases and conditions. The presence of one of these underlying problems often can explain a particular ache. Conversely, aches and pains and arthritis can be the first signs of other problems. Sometimes we don't associate these two seemingly unrelated problems. Diagnosis and treatment of the underlying related condition may correct the associated symptom of pain and arthritis—and sometimes can even be life-saving.

Mrs. S. sought medical help because of a painful foot. The problem was rapidly becoming more severe and interfering with her ability to walk. She saw a podiatrist (foot doctor) and an orthopedist (bone doctor), but neither was able to find a problem. Taking a history of the local pain did not disclose the answer, but on complete physical examination (not limited to her foot), Mrs. S. was found to have a large breast cancer. Her foot pain arose from spread of this problem to the bone. Local x-rays did not reveal the diagnosis, which was confirmed by a bone scan. Unfortunately, the scan also showed several other areas of bone to which the cancer had spread. X-ray treatment resolved the bone pain.

This appendix is designed to help you see how other medical conditions may influence—or even cause—your aches and pains. Certain rheumatologic diseases sometimes also involve other body systems that don't cause aches and pains but that help us identify the disease. Some of these are described in the following pages.

Skin Problems

Many rheumatologic conditions have associated dermatologic or skin problems that can provide clues to the diagnosis.

Lumps under the shin (nodules)

Rheumatoid nodules occur under the skin in less than a fourth of patients with *rheumatoid arthritis.* These people usually have severe and rapidly progressive disease and positive rheumatoid factor blood tests. The nodules are usually found in pressure areas—the elbows, low back, and even the back of the head. They also are often found in the hands. Biopsy can occasionally lead to diagnosis of the arthritis. Rheumatoid arthritis is fully discussed in Chapter 8.

When nodules are seen at the top of the ear, they suggest the presence of gout. These nodules are called *tophi* and are clusters of uric acid crystals. Tophi also occur in the joint space, bursa, and tendon sheaths and can be very destructive. Gout is fully discussed in Chapter 8.

Painful lumps on the shins occur in *erythema nodosum.* This condition is associated with fever, arthritis, muscle pain, and generally feeling ill. The lumps often are associated with underlying infections, especially tuberculosis or fungus infections. Erythema nodosum also occurs with inflammatory bowel disease and *sarcoidosis* and has been linked with use of some drugs, including birth control pills.

Elevated *cholesterol* or *triglycerides (hyperlipidemia)* may cause fatty nodules to appear particularly along tendons. These may imitate the nodules of rheumatoid arthritis or gouty tophi.

Psoriasis

Psoriasis is a common skin disease afflicting as many as 3 percent of the population worldwide. The rash is red with a silvery scale. When the scale is removed, little bleeding points can be seen, which help confirm the diagnosis. Psoriasis usually is found on the elbows and knees but may be found anywhere. Tiny pits may occur in fingernails and toenails. Separation of the nail from its bed with severe scaling also can occur, resulting in crumbling and deformity of the nails. Skin lesions often occur at areas of physical irritation, including trauma, scratching, surgery, or even sunburn. Explosive onset of the psoriasis may even mark the onset of acquired immunodeficiency syndrome (AIDS). However, there are many variations in presentation of this disease and in distribution of lesions over the body.

Some patients with psoriasis have either arthritis or joint aches. The skin lesions do not necessarily occur before the arthritic manifestations and, therefore, the diagnosis isn't always obvious at the onset of arthritis. *Psoriatic arthritis,* the arthritis associated with psoriasis, is classified as one of the enthesopathies or spondyloarthropathies. The onset usually occurs between ages 20 and 50. It seems to affect men and women nearly equally, unlike other related forms of arthritis that more often affect women.

There are several typical patterns of psoriatic arthritis. One causes asymmetric involvement of the fingers and toes. "Sausage" swelling occurs during the acute phase, and the affected joints are immovable. Another type mimics rheumatoid arthritis with more symmetric involvement of joints in the hands and feet but with a negative blood test for rheumatoid factor. In patients with severe nail involvement, the last joint of the fingers may be involved with chronic, though often mild, arthritis.

Arthritis mutilans is the most disabling and mutilating form of arthritis associated with psoriasis. Bony destruction occurs, leading to "pencil in cup" deformities seen on X-ray with telescoping or shortening of the fingers.

The other major form of arthritis associated with psoriasis is spine disease or spondylitis. Most patients with back involvement have the typical HLAB27 surface cell marker found on white blood cells. The disease can start at any point in the spine and often progresses in an almost random fashion.

Reactive Arthritis
(formerly Reiter's Syndrome)

This is another form of spondyloarthropathy or enthesopathy. Most cases last weeks to months but sometimes this can be chronic. It can affect the fingers, toes, heels, low back and other joints. Commonly, the associated arthritis is an inflammation of the tendons and associated joints of the legs as well as a spondylitis or inflammation of the spine. This occurs as a response to having a genitourinary tract or gastrointestinal tract infection by specific bacteria, such as Chlamydia, Campylobacter, Salmonella, Shigella and Yersinia.

Classic Reiter's Syndrome is defined by the triad of arthritis, urethritis, and conjunctivitis—inflammation of the joints, genitals, and eye. Several characteristic skin lesions occur with this disease. The sores resemble psoriasis, with scaly patches.

Other features of classic Reiter's Syndrome include Keratoderma blenorrhagicum, balanitis circinata and mouth ulcers.
Keratoderma blenorrhagicum is a thick yellow scaly rash that usually occurs one or two months after the other symptoms. The rash appears on the soles of the feet and often extends to the toes or other parts of the body. The edges of the eruption have a characteristic circular, scaly border.

Balanitis circinata is the rash that occurs on the penis with Reiter's disease. The scale and crusting lesions coalesce to form a winding pattern on the end of the penis.

Shallow ulcers on the inner surfaces of the mouth also are found with Reiter's syndrome.

Sexually Transmitted Infectious Rashes

Three to fourteen days after venereal contact with the bacteria Neisseria gonorrhoeae, exposed men and women may begin to have signs of infection. Early signs of *gonorrhea* include painful urination and a discharge from the genitals. The disease may spread locally or through the blood. During the blood-borne phase, which occurs in as many as 3 percent of untreated patients, a rash appears. This usually occurs on the tops of the hands and feet as a small number of red bumps. These become blister-like and form pustules that heal in a few weeks. Joint pain involving a number of joints is common, and occasionally an infected, hot, swollen large joint (usually a knee or ankle) is seen. White cells are found in the joint fluid. Bacteria are sometimes also found.

Syphilis can be passed to an unborn child through the mother's infected blood. This infection can lead to bony abnormalities in the infant. In adults, syphilis occurs after direct contact with an infected sore. The infection, caused by the spirochete Treponema pallidum, goes through characteristic stages. The first stage is a chancre or genital ulcer that is painless with raised borders. These ulcers usually occur at the site of contact with the original infection and can also be found in the mouth or anus. The second stage begins about six weeks later in 25 percent of infected patients. It is marked by a diffuse red rash present on all body surfaces, including the palms and soles. Flu-like symptoms often occur, with muscle aches, headache, and sore throat. Temporary hair loss also is common, resulting in a moth-eaten appearance. Hair loss also may involve the beard and eyebrows. Heaped up genital warts, called condylomata lata, may occur around the vaginal lips and anus. In the third or latent phase of the disease, all of the systemic manifestations occur. These include heart and nerve problems. In some cases, the nerve problems are so severe that joint destruction occurs because of lack of sensation. These almost totally destroyed joints are called *Charcot joints* and are typical of late syphilis but can occur with other neurologic diseases as well.

Acquired immunodeficiency syndrome (AIDS) is caused by the Human immunodeficiency virus (HIV) spread through sexual contact or contact with body fluids (for example, from transfusions or shared unsterile needles). About a month after exposure, an acute viral syndrome occurs, with fever, sore throat, diffuse red skin rash and joint and muscle aches and pains. Antibody to the HIV virus is formed over the next year. During this period, lymph nodes enlarge, the white blood cell count drops, and high antibody levels are found. The immune response then decreases and the HIV antibody levels may actually fall. It is at this time that many of the skin signs of the disease are seen. Psoriasis and seborrhea (dandruff) appear to be activated. Because of the impaired immune response, infections are frequent and more dramatic than normal. Viruses cause *shingles,* warts, and even hairy mouth plaques on the tongue. Spread of fungal infections on the skin is common. *Syphilis* appears to progress more rapidly and dramatically when associated with the AIDS virus. About one-third of patients with AIDS will develop a normally unusual skin cancer called Kaposi's sarcoma. This is marked by long purple lesions that occur on all skin surfaces.

Joint manifestations include the early aches and pains, but AIDS may cause a picture nearly identical to *reactive arthritis, rheumatoid arthritis,* or *Sjögren's syndrome.*

Rashes with Viral Infections

Most rashes with viral infections are called "exanthema," which means a diffuse red rash that bursts out or blooms, usually without any scaling.

Rubella or *German Measles* is a contagious viral infection with respiratory spread from infected droplets coughed or sneezed up from an infected carrier. Sometimes called three-day measles, the condition used to be common in children and young adults but now is rare because most children are immunized. After an incubation of two to three weeks, the infected person develops swollen lymph nodes. Headache, fever, and nonspecific aches and pains occur next, followed by the rash. During this period and often for several weeks after the disappearance of the rash, fingers and toes may be painful and swollen.

Erythema infectiosum (also called fifth disease) is a common viral infection caused by a parvovirus that usually occurs in children. The first signs are usually fever, sore throat, itching, and aching after an incubation period of about two to two and a half weeks. A rash in a "slapped cheek" pattern with warmth and red cheeks lasts several days. This then becomes a net-like red rash over the trunk and extremities. Infection with the same virus in adults can lead to diffuse joint pains that may change in location and may last from weeks to years. Infection in pregnant women appears to be associated with increased risk for spontaneous abortion. Researchers have recently linked another type of parvovirus to an arthritis that imitates rheumatoid arthritis.

Infectious mononucleosis is a very common infection caused by the

238

Epstein-Barr virus. In its early stages, "mono" may have a diffuse red skin eruption. After an incubation of one to two months, the disease is marked by fever, sore throat with severe tonsillitis, swollen lymph nodes, and an enlarged spleen, as well as a rash. Hepatitis or inflammation of the liver also may occur. Joint and muscle aches and pains with profound fatigue are common and may last for months.

Kawasaki Syndrome

This disorder, also known as mucocutaneous lymph nodes syndrome, was first described in Japan in the 1960s. It is common in children and has a worldwide distribution. The problem rarely is seen in adults. The condition probably is infectious, but the infecting agent is not known. Skin signs are similar to the viral exanthems with a diffuse red rash over the entire body but primarily in the diaper area. Later the skin over the rash will peel. Lesions in the mouth are an important finding, with red throat and sores around the lips and tongue. The tongue often develops a strawberry appearance. The eyes are usually red. High fevers occur and usually last more than one week. The fevers do not respond to the usual medications and are often very worrisome to parents. Large nontender lymph nodes are found in the neck. Joint pains are common and frank arthritis can develop with painful and swollen joints that may persist for some time. Meningitis or inflammation of the sac around the brain and spinal cord occurs, and death sometimes results from heart and blood vessel complications.

Erythema Chronicum Migrans (Lyme Disease)

This infection, transmitted by the bite of a deer tick, causes a flu-like illness with muscle and joint aches and pains, fatigue, headache, low-grade fever, and (usually but not always) a typical rash. The rash is an expanding area of redness with central clearing. Onset is usually at the site of the tick bite. Similar secondary lesions, smaller in size, may later develop over the body. The outer border of the lesions is usually bright red and flat, although it occasionally may be slightly raised.

The second stage of the disease can include heart and nerve

complications. The third stage, which may develop months to years after the tick bite, is characterized by episodic arthritis involving one or many joints and possibly migrating from one area to another. These latter stages do not have skin manifestations. More information on Lyme disease can be found elsewhere in this book.

Periodontal Disease and Rheumatoid Arthritis

There have been several recent studies linking periodontal (gum) disease and rheumatoid arthritis. It is uncertain if the cause is bacteria in the gums or simply inflammation of the gums. Another smaller study suggests that treating the periodontal disease may mitigate existing rheumatoid arthritis.

All of this should not be surprising since we know that certain infections are linked to chronic arthritis and that even a bacteria H. pylori is a cause of peptic ulcer disease.
There is definitely more to come on this topic in the near future!

Drug-Related Skin Reactions

Medications sometimes cause rashes. The most typical patterns include a diffuse red rash over the entire body, with flat, itching plaques called urticaria or hives. Peeling rashes and large blistering rashes can occur, as well as rashes brought out by sun exposure. Some of these drug-induced rashes are associated with other allergic manifestations including difficulty breathing and even severe joint pains. Rashes can last a long time but usually resolve quickly when the offending medication is withdrawn. Thiazide diuretics (water pills), tetracycline derivatives, and sulfa drugs are common causes of rashes. Anti-inflammatory arthritis medications and methotrexate, used to treat some forms of arthritis, have also been implicated. Many other drugs also can cause rashes.

Medications can also activate a group of conditions called *porphyria*. With this disorder, abnormal production of blood protein causes various abnormal chemicals called porphyrins to accumulate in the blood, urine, feces, and tissues. Porphyrins have a red-brown pigmentation and absorb specific wave lengths of light that can damage the skin. Symptoms include typical pigment changes and blistering rashes, particularly on sun-exposed skin. Alcohol, barbiturates, sulfa drugs, estrogens, and even stress or starvation can cause forms of the disease. In some cases, there is marked skin pain and tenderness. The acute forms are associated with intense abdominal pain, seizures, weakness, and confusion.

Follow the directions in chapter 11 to learn if any medications you are taking are likely to cause these problems.

Lupus Rashes

Almost 90 percent of patients with *systemic lupus erythematosus* have one or more skin signs that help establish the diagnosis. Probably the most common is a rash in a "butterfly" distribution over the cheeks and nose, but sparing the skin folds around the lips and mouth. This "malar" rash characteristic of systemic lupus is discussed more fully in chapter 8.

Discoid lupus lesions also can occur with systemic lupus but also can occur independently without other features of the systemic disease. These lesions are red and raised initially and will scar. They often progress to depressed scars with plugging around the hair follicles. Lesions in the scalp cause patchy baldness with scarring. Discoid lesions also can occur after sun exposure or trauma.

Mouth ulcers also are a clue to the diagnosis of systemic disease, as are rashes following exposure to sunlight.

Raynaud's phenomenon, enlarged skin veins, scarring and non-scarring balding, and vasculitis-associated skin lesions also are common with systemic lupus.

A third type of lupus, called *subacute cutaneous lupus,* causes a non-scarring group of skin rashes that mainly occur on the trunk. Lesions usually are flat, red, irregular plates covered with scale. Also, a pattern of converging small red bumps occurs on sun-exposed areas. The lesions can last a long time but usually heal without scarring. These patients usually have a characteristic antibody (called anti-Ro or SSA). So-called neonatal lupus can occur in infants born to women with this disorder. The infants usually have a rash similar to the mother's but also have a high incidence of congenital heart block, a dangerous situation in which the electrical system in the heart is not functioning.

Sun-Caused Rashes

Medications taken orally, injected, or applied to the skin can cause sensitivity to the sun. This "phototoxicity" is manifested by redness and, later, pigment changes in the exposed areas. The reaction subsides when the drug is withdrawn. Medication reactions are sometimes associated with transient joint aches and pains.

Sun-related rashes are one of the diagnostic clues for *systemic lupus erythematosus.* In some people, the sun can cause a flare of either the form of lupus limited to the skin or the systemic disease. Sun-related rashes also may occur with other connective tissues diseases, particularly *mixed connective tissue disease* and *scleroderma.*

Scleroderma

In all forms of this disorder, connective tissue is damaged, first with inflammation and degenerative changes and then with intense fibrosis. This fibrosis causes the stiffness noted in the skin and internal organs. Scleroderma can occur in a localized form (with changes limited to the skin) or in more generalized forms.

Morphea is one type of limited scleroderma. It occurs most commonly in middle-aged women and starts with one or more raised purple patches on the skin. With "healing," the center of the patch becomes scarred and hard. It is elevated with a persistent red-purple border.

Linear scleroderma also is a limited form of the disease. The long bands of thickened skin may extend deeper and involve muscle and other underlying structures. Joints may develop contractures or permanent bends. This form of the disease clearly interferes with joint and muscle function.

A rare form of localized disease is "en coup de sabre," which indeed looks like the cut of a sword. With this form, there is a scar-like fibrotic band, usually down the face but occurring elsewhere on the body as well. Skin atrophy occurs, leaving the appearance of injury.

Generalized scleroderma or progressive systemic sclerosis initially involves primarily the skin and is slowly progressive but at times can advance rapidly and be fatal. The disease usually begins with skin changes. In most cases, the first symptoms are a reversible blood vessel spasm in the fingers and toes called *Raynaud's phenomenon.* Severe and recurrent attacks cause scarring with ulceration and pitting of the fingertips. The skin itself first swells, causing sausage swelling of the fingers and toes and a tight, mask-like face. Swelling is then replaced by tough, bound-down skin. The tightening and binding down of the skin over the fingers leads to an inability to straighten the fingers, resulting in a claw hand covered with tough, tight skin. This change is called sclerodactyly. Further binding down of the skin causes a tapered pointy appearance of the fingertips and actually leads to disappearance of the bone in the fingertips. *Telangiectasias* (surface dilation of tiny blood vessels called capillaries) occur primarily over the face and hands. Early in the disease, telangiectasias are seen at the fingernail bed.

Patients with scleroderma typically complain of joint and muscle pain, as well as weakness. A frank inflammatory process may occur in the muscle in active disease. Involvement of the esophagus commonly causes difficulty with swallowing. Dilation of the bowel and lack of movement also occurs in the intestines and leads to a characteristic X-ray picture. Patients may develop poor intestinal absorption of foodstuffs. Constipation is common because of loss of bowel motility. Lung disease occurs from loss of elasticity of the lungs. Oxygen crosses the lung tissue into the blood less efficiently. Heart problems also stem from fibrosis or scarring of the heart muscle or from the lung problem. Not only is the pump function of the heart itself impaired, but changes in conduction of electrical impulses in the heart cause

243

disturbances in rhythm. The kidney involvement leads to potentially severe hypertension (high blood pressure), which does not respond to treatment. The kidneys lose the ability to filter out waste products, which then accumulate in the blood.

CREST syndrome is a more limited and perhaps less severe form of the disease. One criterion for the diagnosis is calcinosis or calcium deposits under the skin. Raynaud's and esophagus abnormalities are other criteria. Sclerodactyly described above with tightening and tapering of the fingertips is still another. Telangiectasias are enlargement of normally tiny blood vessels that can form a red or purple netlike pattern the skin. The presence of telangiectasias is the last criterion for CREST syndrome. This limited variant but may be associated within the blood vessels in the lungs. This increased pressure is termed pulmonary hypertension.

Fasciitis

The fascia is a tough tissue that lies beneath the skin. It can become inflamed in certain conditions. Some of these can be confused with early *scleroderma. Eosinophilic fasciitis* occurs more often in young men after prolonged exercise. It begins with painful and tender swelling of the arms and legs. With time, these areas become indurated, which leads to confusion with scleroderma. However, the induration has a more irregular texture with puckering that gives the skin an "orange-peel" appearance. Other findings are fever, fatigue, and weight loss. Joint pains are common. Diagnosis is made by a deep biopsy, including the fascia and muscle. Laboratory tests are helpful because there is an increase in blood eosinophils (a type of white blood cell).

Toxic exposures have also produced similar skin problems. Rapeseed oil has caused a syndrome of headache, fluid in the lungs, muscle aches, increased blood eosinophils, and a rash progressing to late nerve damage with typical scleroderma-like skin changes. This is called *toxic oil syndrome.* It is believed that blood vessel injury by the rapeseed oil was the cause.

A number of other medications and industrial chemicals may produce inflammation and thickening of the fascia, producing a picture similar to scleroderma. These chemicals include *polyvinyl chlorides* (used in industry), some drugs used as chemotherapy, and *L-tryptophan,* which until recently was commonly used as a nonprescription drug to help people sleep. Silicone breast implants have been implicated by some as a rare cause of a scleroderma-like condition but this is quite controversial.

Telangiectasias

Telangiectasias are areas of enlarged blood vessels seen on the skin. They may look like a fine web or like a more generalized redness. They usually occur over the face. On the hands, they give a characteristic redness to the palms and can also be visualized as dilated, hairpin loops of capillaries at the base of the fingernails. Telangiectasias are common with *systemic lupus, mixed connective tissue disease, dermatomyositis,* and *progressive systemic sclerosis (scleroderma)* or the more limited form of scleroderma called *CREST syndrome.* These telangiectasias occur as extensive flat mats usually on the face, especially around the lips, and on the hands. The appearance of these dime-sized mats is unique to this family of connective tissue disorders and is one of the diagnostic criteria. Association of telangiectasias with aches and pains should suggest the possibility of one of these systemic diseases.

Telangiectasias often occur in other circumstances as well. Conditions of excess estrogen, including use of birth control medication, are associated with increased formation of "spiders" or telangiectasias. They often occur at the site of skin damage by the sun. Steroids by mouth or even overuse of steroid creams can also injure the skin, causing thinning and telangiectasias, often with easy bruising. Telangiectasias are found on the surface of a basal cell skin cancer and may also occur with some birth defects that affect skin and nerves. With *Osler- Weber-Rendu disease,* these blood vessel deformities can be associated with excess bleeding of the nose and intestinal tract.

Calcium Deposits in the Skin

Calcinosis or calcium deposits in the skin occur in several rheumatologic diseases and may be important in diagnosis. Calcinosis is one of the diagnostic criteria for the form of *scleroderma* called CREST *syndrome.* CREST is an acronym for calcinosis, Raynaud's phenomenon, esophagus problems, sclerodactyly (finger narrowing), and telangiectasias. Calcium deposits usually occur in the tips of the fingers. They can also occur over other bony prominences, including the knees and elbows. The deposits are hard, usually small whitish nodules. The surrounding skin can often become red, hot, and irritated, especially when a nodule breaks and disgorges its contents to the surface of the skin. The other features of this disease are fully discussed under scleroderma or progressive systemic sclerosis.

Deeper blood vessel calcifications are commonly seen in individuals with diabetes.

Dermatomyositis

Dermatomyositis is a disease of children and older adults. It is a disease of muscle (myo-) inflammation (itis), which is associated with typical skin signs. With this disease, there is muscle weakness and destruction with release of muscle enzymes into the blood where they can be measured. Electrical impulses from the damaged muscle also are altered and can be detected by the electromyogram. Muscle biopsies also reflect inflammatory changes in the muscle.

The most characteristic skin feature of dermatomyositis is the heliotrope or purple discoloration around the eyes. Violet to red rashes with scaling also occurs, first in a patchy form, usually in sun-exposed form. The skin changes are usually very pronounced over the knuckles of the hands. With sun exposure, the rash usually intensifies in color and may become bright red. Another skin manifestation is Gottron's papules, which are small flat rashes over the knuckles and sides of the fingers. Redness and dilated capillaries at the base of the nails are another hallmark of this process. In some cases, this disease has been associated with an increased risk of cancer.

Polymyositis (a form *of myositis)* is the name for the disease in which the muscles are inflamed but no skin involvement is noted.

Vitiligo is an acquired loss of pigment that can begin at any age but usually occurs in adults. The skin develops a very patchy coloration that can be disfiguring to the dark-skinned individual. Vitiligo appears to be an autoimmune problem with antibodies causing destruction of the melanocytes or pigment cells in the skin. Areas of trauma and sun damage are particularly likely to develop these under-pigmented patches. Vitiligo is commonly associated with connective tissue diseases, such as systemic lupus erythematosus, mixed connective tissue disease, myositis, and progressive systemic sclerosis (scleroderma). It is also associated with other autoimmune mediated diseases including diabetes, pernicious anemia, and thyroid disease. As many as a third of patients with vitiligo will have thyroid disease.

Panniculitis or Inflammation of the Fat Layer

Nodular panniculitis is a rare group of disorders with inflammation and destruction of the fatty layer under the skin. This condition often is associated with joint and muscle pain. Abdominal pain, sometimes with an enlarged spleen and liver, is occasionally found. One group of these disorders is associated with underlying disease of the pancreas, often alcohol-induced, but also with hidden cancer. *Erythema nodosum* sometimes is included in this group. Panniculitis occurs in *Weber-Christian disease* and may occasionally occur in *lupus.*

Infections

Bacterial Infections of the Bone (Osteomyelitis) Osteomyelitis is an infection of the bone. The thigh and foot are most commonly involved. The bone may become infected after a penetrating wound resulting in skin infection. This often happens when we step on something sharp. Intravenous drug abuse is another cause of bone infection.

Bone can be infected by any blood-borne organism. This happens most often in children and may involve more than one area. The very elderly also are susceptible and can have infections of the spine. Diabetics or people with other blood vessel diseases seem to be particularly prone to osteomyelitis. Local ulcers or sores on the feet provide another site for infection. Sickle cell disease also predisposes to osteomyelitis.

Acute osteomyelitis is usually accompanied by fever, chills, and a high white count, with local pain, tenderness, redness, and swelling. Blood cultures often show bacteria in the blood. Even with treatment with antibiotics, some of these infections are not cured and become chronic. Delayed treatment contributes to this risk. Chronic infections are very resistant to treatment. Recurrent bouts may occur years apart. Local tenderness and drainage to the skin are common.

Gonorrhea

Gonorrhea is the most common cause of infectious arthritis in sexually active young adults. The infecting bacterium is spread through sexual contact. In the earliest phase of the disease, there is a characteristic flat red rash that often becomes pustular. At times the infecting organism can be cultured from these pustules. The rash usually occurs on the body, arms, and legs but may also involve the palms and soles. Joint aches are common in this phase. The second phase involves frank arthritis of one or more of the joints, including the hips and knees. Most of the time, the tendons are also painfully involved with local swelling and tenderness. This is likely to occur at the ankles, wrists, and hands but it may also involve the lower extremity joints and tendons.

Lyme Disease

This infection is transmitted by the deer tick. The infecting organism is called a spirochete and is distantly related to the spirochete causing *syphilis*. In both these diseases, a prolonged infection persists with symptoms sometimes occurring many years after the initial infection.

Because deer ticks carry the bacteria, people with this disease usually have a history of being outdoors, perhaps hunting, gardening or even playing golf, in an area where the disease occurs. Most cases in the United States are found in the Northeast, especially in Massachusetts, Connecticut, New York, and New Jersey, as well as in the northern Midwest states and the far west.

The disease has three stages. Stage I occurs within a month of infection. A characteristic rash with irregular red borders and central clearing occurs. Unfortunately, this unique and characteristic rash isn't always present. Other early signs are nonspecific, such as low-grade fever, chills, fatigue, headaches, sore throat, and muscle and joint aches and pains.

Stage II is marked by nerve symptoms. Severe headaches and stiff neck occur with inflammation of the brain and meninges (the sac surrounding the central nervous system). Cranial nerve involvement such as Bell's palsy (weakness of the facial nerve) and peripheral neuropathies may occur. Involvement of the heart, especially complete heart block, also occurs at this stage.

Arthritis develops in Stage II. It is asymmetric, usually involving one or a few joints. Large joints, especially the ankles and knees, are most commonly involved, though small joints can also be affected. Occasionally a symmetric involvement of the small joints (hand, wrist) occurs, mimicking *rheumatoid arthritis. Myositis* (muscle inflammation) may occur. There are periods of spontaneous remission with frequent recurrences. It is often this sporadic pattern of arthritis associated with heart and nerve findings that provides the clue to diagnosis of this disease. Chronic recurrences can lead to permanent erosions and joint destruction.

Hand involvement also is seen late in the disease and is associated with late skin rash over the fingers. This can progress to bone and joint changes.

Acquired Immunodeficiency Syndrome (AIDS)

Infection with HIV or human immunodeficiency virus is the cause of acquired immunodeficiency syndrome (AIDS). The disease usually is spread by sexual contact but also can be spread by contact with other body fluids, particularly blood. Spread can be by transfusion or use of shared needles or nonsterile surgical or dental equipment. In addition to people with diagnosed AIDS, there are many asymptomatic carriers, each of whom is capable of spreading the virus.

The first sign of infection is usually a typical viral syndrome that occurs about three to twelve weeks after infection. Initial symptoms last about two weeks and include joint and muscle aches and pain with low-grade fever, sore throat, headaches, enlarged lymph nodes, fatigue, and skin rash. A change in ratio of infection-fighting cells (called T cells) occurs at this time. Some people who are exposed to the virus appear to develop a prolonged initial phase with continued lymph node enlargement and aches and pains. This has been termed AIDS-related complex (ARC) and is thought to be another form of the early infection.

Antibodies eventually form in response to the HIV virus. They usually are evident within a few months of infection but may not form for more than three years. Tests commonly used to detect AIDS currently depend on the presence of antibodies. Other tests detect the virus itself or its antigens (proteins). It is possible to spread the disease while the AIDS test is still negative, before any antibody is made. Therefore, even a negative AIDS test doesn't ensure a person against having AIDS or giving AIDS to others.

Some proportion of people with HIV progress to the full syndrome. The normal mechanisms the body uses for fighting infections and malignancies (cancers) are destroyed, and AIDS patients are subject to many infections, including infections of the joints and bones (osteomyelitis). In addition, malignancies, especially Kaposi's sarcoma, are increased. Immune deregulation also causes an increase in other antibodies, including autoantibodies seen in systemic lupus, rheumatoid arthritis, and other autoimmune-mediated diseases. The virus also directly injures the central nervous system. AIDS dementia with confusion, behavioral changes, and even changes in movement occur. Peripheral neuropathy can also occur with numbness, weakness, and abnormal sensations of the arms and legs. Other manifestations include decreased gastric acid secretion and malabsorption of nutrients. Kidney problems develop, and the heart muscle is injured. Severe joint pains can occur, particularly in the lower extremities. *Reactive arthritis* has been identified frequently in HIV infected people, as has *psoriatic arthritis,* primarily involving the lower extremities and spine. A syndrome resembling *rheumatoid arthritis* has also been seen with arthritis primarily involving the hands and feet. In addition, a syndrome similar to *Sjögren's syndrome* may occur. Muscle disease *(myopathy)* including *myositis* (inflamed muscle) may occur. A variety of forms *of vasculitis* (blood vessel inflammation) has been described.

Thankfully, combination antiviral medication treatment regimens have changed this previously devastating disease into a more chronic condition in most cases.

Shingles

Shingles is an infection caused by the herpes varicella zoster virus, the same virus that causes chicken pox. After infection, virus particles seem to remain in the nerve roots of the spine. If the immune system is suppressed, the virus may once again multiply and spread along the nerve root. This causes a line of tiny blebs called vesicles, which are usually on a red base. The area along the route becomes sensitive to touch, and pain can be very sharp and severe. With time, the rash forms scabs and heals but often leaves a scar. The shingles rash almost always is on only one side of the body and in a line. Early detection and treatment are important. Eye involvement can lead to blindness.

Tuberculosis

Most of us think of tuberculosis as a disease of the lung, with cough and weight loss, usually affecting the poor. However, tuberculosis can involve bones and joints and may affect the spine, particularly the mid to low back, hips, and knees. Tuberculosis also can affect wrists and elbows. Usually only one joint is affected, but more than one can be involved. Active lung disease is not always present with bone or joint involvement. Tuberculosis can affect the bones directly, causing osteomyelitis (bone infections).

Thankfully, tuberculosis of bones occurs in less than 1 percent of all new cases of tuberculosis. Still it should be kept in mind when joint involvement occurs. Tuberculosis has been known to cause *carpal tunnel syndrome* (compression of the median nerve at the wrist).

The Yeast Connection

The theoretic basis of the yeast connection is that the common yeast, Candida albicans, produces toxins that cause a type of allergic reaction within the body. Among symptoms attributed to Candida hypersensitivity are fatigue, headache, anxiety, mood swings, poor memory, dizziness, insomnia, itching, muscle aches, muscle weakness, joint pain, postnasal drip, sore throat, cough, chest pain, shortness of breath, bloating, belching, heartburn, diarrhea, constipation, impotence, and others. However, no controlled studies have showed that sensitivity to Candida causes such a myriad of symptoms. The connections are believed to be unproven by the American Academy of Immunology.

It is possible that Candida plays a role—although probably a limited role—in some illnesses. Until more evidence is gathered, however, it cannot be concluded that Candida hypersensitivity is a distinct cause of chronic fatigue.

Post polio Syndrome

Individuals who had polio during childhood or adolescence sometimes develop muscle problems 25 to 30 years later. However, all other causes of muscle problems need to be excluded—including orthopedic problems such as fractures or degenerative arthritis, stroke, nerve damage, or depression.

In acute poliomyelitis, the nerves are attacked by a virus and many nerve cells are killed. These cells connect to muscle fibers and regulate movement. When the nerve cells are infected, the nerve path to the brain is interrupted and messages can't get through. The muscle becomes paralyzed. However, a large number of infected cells will recover, and new nerve connections grow between the muscles and uninjured or recovering nerve cells. These new connections once again allow the patients to control muscles.

The post polio syndrome seems to be a late destruction occurring in previously damaged areas. Recent research suggests that the recurrence of muscle weakness is due to either persistence or recurrence of the polio infection.

In post polio syndrome, new muscle weakness and loss of size in previously affected muscle occurs. Deformity may also increase in areas of weakness. Spinal curvatures or twisting of limbs may be evident. Muscle pain and fine tremors may be associated. Difficulty with swallowing and breathing also may occur. Periods of decreased breathing during sleep (sleep apnea) are found, and severe fatigue usually is a problem. Symptoms may worsen over time, sometimes slowly but sometimes rapidly.

Treatment is generally limited to supportive measures. Physical therapy with a carefully designed exercise program is a must.

Infectious Arthritis

Sudden swelling, redness, pain, and immobility may signal an acute infection in the joint. Infection is one of the few emergency causes of arthritis because when this is not diagnosed and treated rapidly, permanent joint damage will occur. Rapid treatment with antibiotics and removal of the infected joint fluid often cures the problem and preserves joint function.

Bacterial infectious arthritis usually involves only one joint, although sometimes it affects several joints. Onset of pain, redness, swelling, and stiffness usually is sudden. Most often large joints, such as the hip and knee, are involved, but the shoulder, elbow, wrist, and ankle also may be affected. In some cases, a rash and migrating joint aches and pains may appear early. High fever and chills occur with infections caused by bacteria in the blood (sepsis). Sometimes a joint infection will develop after a penetrating injury.

Subacute bacterial endocarditis (SBE) is infection of the heart, usually caused by a bacteria present in the mouth called streptococcus. Other bacteria may be responsible as well. Usually, an abnormal heart valve becomes infected with the organism due to the bacteria gaining entrance to the blood during a dental procedure. This may also occur via other portals of entrance into the blood such as a urinary tract infection. This infection is a relatively slow in progression and can lead to fever, fatigue, excessive sweating, weakness and a feeling of malaise (feeling ill at ease). In addition, it may cause joint and tendon sheath inflammation (arthritis and tenosynovitis, respectively). It is diagnosed by blood cultures and echocardiographic evaluation of the heart valves. High dose antibiotic treatment for at least four weeks is the preferred treatment. SBE may lead to permanent heart valve damage if not treated early enough. Subacute bacterial endocarditis clearly may mimic inflammatory arthritis.

Specific joint infections have been discussed in other sections of the book. *Lyme arthritis* is caused by an organism carried by the deer tick. Illness starts with flu-like symptoms with aches and pains, low-grade fever, fatigue, headache, and a characteristic rash with an irregular, growing, red border with central clearing. Later stages may include frank arthritis, which usually affects the large joints, especially the knees, but can also mimic *rheumatoid arthritis* with involvement of both large and small joints, including the hands. Bacteria can be found in the joint space. Nervous system and heart involvement can occur late in the disease.

In young, sexually active adults, *gonorrhea* is the most common cause of acute arthritis, usually involving one or two joints, especially wrists, knees, or ankles. Joint inflammation of the tendon sheaths (called tenosynovitis) often involves the fingers, wrists, toes, and ankles. The disease usually is spread by sexual contact. The early phase is marked with a flat, red rash that may become pustular. The rash is often on the arms or legs. Generalized aches and pains in the joints are common in the early phase.

Syphilis is another sexually transmitted bacterial infection that causes joint symptoms, although most of its joint manifestations occur after the acute infection. *Reactive arthritis* or *Reiter's syndrome* also is a post infectious arthritis.

Staphylococcal infections usually start from the skin. The organism normally lives on the skin and causes problems only when it enters the body. The organism can enter through dirty needles cuts, or skin wounds. The organism is then carried by the blood, leading to local areas of infection. When joints are involved, a rapidly damaging arthritis occurs. This is a medical emergency and needs rapid treatment to avoid permanent joint damage. Staph commonly involves the knee or hip, although other joints can be involved.

Staphylococcal arthritis should be suspected in patients with known blood-borne infection. Important predisposing factors include severe skin infections and intravenous drug addiction. Joint infections can be diagnosed by sampling the joint fluid and testing for infection. Treatment includes antibiotics and repeated removal of joint fluid by needle or surgical drainage. Staph is also a leading cause of infection in artificial joints. When it occurs, the prosthetic joint usually must be removed. Replacement usually is delayed until a prolonged course of antibiotics is administered; new joints may have a higher infection rate than normal.

Acute rheumatic fever is associated with arthritis but is not really a joint infection. It is a post infectious arthritis that occurs after an infection, usually a sore throat, with certain members of the Streptococcus family.

Other bacterial infections of the joints are more unusual. Many occur in people with impaired immune responses such as AIDS patients. Infections with the more unusual gram-negative bacteria also occur with certain diseases. Youngsters with *sickle cell disease* often have *Salmonella infections*. Newborns and the very elderly seem more susceptible to E. coli infections. Very young children seem to have a high rate of infection with H. influenzae, which most often causes hip infections.

Tuberculosis can cause infectious arthritis. The weight-bearing areas, especially the knees and hips, are most often affected. The spine may become involved, usually in the mid or upper back. This infection is called

Pott's disease and often causes a deformity of the back with an unusually pronounced curvature.

In some parts of the United States, certain fungal infections can affect the joints. *Coccidioidomycosis* usually involves the knee. *Blastomycosis* may affect knees, ankles, or elbows. *Sporotrichosis* is a fungal infection usually seen in gardeners and is sometimes contracted from the thorn of the rose. It can infect skin and tendons and can involve the joints.

Many viral infections also affect joints. *Hepatitis* is one and can occur in at least three different forms—hepatitis A, B, and C. All have a flu-like pattern with fever, nausea, profound fatigue, rashes, aches, and pains. Severe joint pains in small joints of the hands as well as wrists, elbows, shoulders and knees may occur, particularly with hepatitis B. After this early stage, abnormalities of liver function are found, often with jaundice. Hepatitis B may lead to a chronic infection in some people, with persistent joint pains.

Respiratory Diseases

Pleurisy

Pleurisy is simply inflammation of the sac that surrounds the lungs. The symptoms are primarily severe, sharp chest pain that varies in intensity with position and with breathing. Fluid may enter into this space around the lungs, producing what is called "pleural effusion."

Pleurisy, often associated with serositis (inflammation of the sac surrounding the heart and intestines), is one of the diagnostic criteria of *systemic lupus erythematosus.* While lupus cells (white cells that have engulfed a red cell) are no longer used as a major diagnostic test for systemic lupus, their presence in a pleural effusion strongly suggests lupus as the diagnosis.

Pleurisy also is associated with other autoimmune diseases including *mixed connective tissue disease* and *rheumatoid arthritis.*

See discussion elsewhere in the book.

Blood Diseases

Anemia
(Decrease in Red Blood Cells)

Anemia is the general term for a decrease in the red blood cells in the body. This also means a decrease in hemoglobin—the substance in the blood responsible for carrying oxygen to the tissues. Basically the condition can arise in two ways: First, by improper production of hemoglobin or blood cells and, second, by loss of blood cell mass with bleeding or destruction of red cells. Improper production of hemoglobin or blood cells is associated with many rheumatologic diseases as well as other conditions that can lead to aches and pains. Hemolysis, or the destruction of red cells, also is associated with several rheumatologic conditions.

Pernicious anemia is the result of inability to properly absorb *vitamin* B12 from dietary sources. This is an autoimmune disease that usually occurs because of a deficiency of intrinsic factor. Intrinsic factor is secreted by cells in the stomach lining and helps in the absorption of vitamin B12 from the gut into the body. In addition to anemia, deficiency of vitamin B12 is associated with severe nerve problems. Dementia or changes in thinking may occur. Low vitamin B12 levels are associated with sensation changes including nerve pain. Low vitamin B12 levels may also cause severe fatigue.

Anemia may also occur because of genetically determined abnormal production of blood. The most well-known of these anemias is *sickle cell anemia*. Because of the incorrect incorporation of one amino acid into the hemoglobin molecule (essentially one link in a long chain), the entire function of the molecule is altered and the cell actually changes shape. These "sickled cells" tend to cause sludging that can lead to severe bone pain. Patients sometimes have severe hip

257

pain because of *aseptic necrosis,* or destruction, in the hip. The destruction is caused by poor blood flow. *Osteomyelitis* or bone infection also may occur with sickle-cell anemia.

Anemia is one of the criteria for diagnosis of *systemic lupus erythematosus.* So-called anemia of chronic disease is commonly associated with *rheumatoid arthritis.* Also, flares of arthritis are often marked by a worsening of the anemia.

Abnormal Platelet Count

Platelets are very small cells in the blood that clump together in the blood vessel to form a clot after injury. This helps stop bleeding from a cut or broken vessel.

A low platelet count *(thrombocytopenia)* is one of the criteria for diagnosing *systemic lupus erythematosus (lupus).* With thrombocytopenia, platelets usually function normally and there is no significant bleeding unless the platelet count is extremely low. Sometimes, however, there is trouble with continued blood flow, often after delivery of a child. Oozing under the skin also may occur, causing bruise-like skin lesions.

Low platelet counts also occur in *idiopathic thrombocytopenic* purpura (ITP). With this disease, platelets are destroyed by antibodies. Frequently this diagnosis is made and then, sometime later, the other criteria for lupus become obvious. Therefore, it is usually prudent to look for lupus when ITP is diagnosed.

High platelet counts *(thrombocytosis)* occur with chronic bleeding as seen in a colon cancer, but they will also occur with inflammation in general. It is very common to see a patient with *rheumatoid arthritis* with a very high platelet count. High platelet counts may be seen in *sarcoidosis.* Infection and malignancy (cancer) can also be associated with high platelet counts. Elevated platelet counts may be, but are not always, associated with disorders of increased clotting or thrombosis.

Venous thrombosis (clots in veins) or *thrombophlebitis* (inflamed veins with clots) occur most often after immobilization—either with prolonged sitting as on a long trip or when bedridden. It usually occurs in the legs and causes swelling and pain, particularly in the calf. Pain behind the knee also may occur. Deep vein thrombophlebitis also is often associated with pain in the thigh.

Venous thrombosis can also be associated with cancer. This phenomenon is called *Trousseau's syndrome.* The thrombosis can occur in a variety of locations and may occur in the arms as well as the legs. The thrombosis often occurs before the tumor is diagnosed. Sometimes even the arteries develop clots in Trousseau's syndrome.

Increased clotting is also often seen in *systemic lupus erythematosus.* A misnamed "lupus anticoagulant" is associated with abnormal blood clotting. It may lead to an increased tendency to form clots or a tendency to bleed. Lupus also can lower the platelet count, causing easy bruising and bleeding.

Hemophilia and other related disorders are caused by an inherited lack of one of the protein factors required for normal clotting. Repeated bleeding into a joint can cause destruction, such as might occur as a child begins to walk and frequently falls. Larger joints, especially the weight-bearing joints of the legs, are most often involved.

Nerve Conditions
Headaches

Classic *migraine headaches* come and go. They occur more often in women and usually during middle age. They usually begin with abnormal sensations, including visual symptoms. Facial tingling and numbness are common, and visual changes range from haziness or shimmering to distinct areas of visual loss. These symptoms then

259

disappear and are replaced by a severe headache that is described as throbbing or pounding. The headache often is only on one side and may be felt over the eye but may become generalized. It is often accompanied by nausea and vomiting. Light sensitivity frequently is described.

Temporal or *giant cell arteritis* is an inflammatory vasculitis causing headache and visual disturbances with potential blindness in elderly patients. There is usually tenderness over the temporal artery as well as more generalized scalp tenderness. Jaw pain may occur during chewing. This disorder requires emergency care and is discussed fully earlier in the book

Glaucoma is another cause of headache and blindness in elderly patients. Increased pressure in the globe of the eye leads to severe pain and visual loss. Acute glaucoma may also be accompanied by nausea and vomiting. The eye is usually red and tender and feels rock-hard. This is a medical emergency and needs the immediate attention of an ophthalmologist.

Tension headaches appear to be most prominent at times of stress. The pain is steady and often described as a tightness or pressure, sometimes vice-like. The pain usually is located at the front of the head but may occur in back where the neck muscles attach to the skull. The onset of pain is gradual and appears to be worse at the end of the day and may be relieved by relaxing or massaging the back of the neck. The headaches usually last for hours but sometimes last for days.

Sinus headaches are generally located in the facial area, usually directly over the involved sinuses. The affected areas may be tender. Headaches are recurrent and appear to change with position. Generally they are worse when lying down and improve on arising from bed in the morning. Involvement of the sinuses may be due to allergy or to drainage problems—either of which can lead to sinus infection. Rarely, blood vessel inflammation called *Wegener's granulomatosis* involves the sinuses, causing similar symptoms.

Periodic Limb Movement Disorder (PLMD)

This poorly understood malady is related to *Restless Legs Syndrome (RLS)*. Most people with RLS have PLMD but the opposite is not true. In PLMD the arms and legs move involuntarily while asleep. In RLS, the movements occur while awake and when asleep. Patients with PLMD have a difficult time staying and falling asleep and are tired during the day. The limb movements occur during the first half of the night in non-REM (rapid eye movement) sleep. PLMD is common, occurring in about 4% of adults. It may be associated with obstructive sleep apnea, diabetes, and iron deficiency. A sleep study will help make the diagnosis.

A variety of treatments been used. Some of these treatments are identical to those used in Parkinson's disease.

Other medications that are tried include clonazepam, diazepam, bupropion, and melatonin.

Tic Douloureux

This disorder is also called *trigeminal neuralgia*. In this condition, the patient suffers from episodes of severe, sharp, and piercing pain on one side of the face, often near the jaw. The cause is unknown. It usually occurs in older patients, and pain can be triggered by even lightly touching a sensitive area, brushing the teeth, or chewing. The pain can be excruciating, and the episodes are usually of short duration. Many episodes can occur daily, however.

Other conditions that can cause similar pain include shingles, certain neurologic conditions, tumors, and migraines. Tic douloureux is usually treated with medications that often are quite effective. For refractory cases, surgery might be indicated and may be helpful.

Endocrine and Metabolic Diseases

Diabetes Mellitus

This is a common disease caused by faulty glucose metabolism. One form usually begins in childhood and requires insulin injections. This may be an autoimmune disorder. Another form occurs later in life and often can be controlled with diet and oral medication. Insulin is sometimes required for the adult-onset form of diabetes.

Diabetics have many forms of arthritis and the incidence of all forms appears to be higher than in the general population. This may be because abnormal sugar metabolism damages the cartilage, making it more susceptible to osteoarthritis and to the deposition of calcium in the joint space. Deposition of uric acid crystals in the joint space causing gout is also more common in diabetics.

Diabetes often injures small blood vessels. When these vessels are part of the blood supply to the nerves, abnormalities in sensation occur. This damage results in a *peripheral neuropathy* that can cause numbness, tingling, loss of position sense, and diminished recognition of painful stimuli. Because of this, the joints may be subject to repetitive trauma and can become injured. This leads to a characteristic form of degenerative arthritis called the *Charcot joint,* which also occurs with other causes of nerve injury. This form of joint destruction occurs in the feet and knees. Diabetic nerve injuries also cause sensations of severe pain without any apparent external cause, usually in the feet.

Diabetics may also have injury to other nerves, with numbness and tingling and sometimes loss of function. An example is *carpal tunnel syndrome,* which causes hand and wrist pain that can ascend up the arm. *Meralgia paresthetica* causes severe burning pain on the outside of the thigh with a loss of sensation. *Femoral neuropathy* may cause severe pain in the front and outside aspect of the thigh. Diabetic involvement of the nerves controlling eye movement may cause double vision (crossed eyes).

Diabetics also may have reduced resistance to infection. Because of this, joint and bone infections *(osteomyelitis)* may be more common. Infections caused by unusual organisms also tend to be somewhat more common with diabetes. Care must be taken to provide broad antibiotic protection if the exact cause of an illness is not known.

Thyroid Disease

Thyroid hormone is secreted by the thyroid gland in the neck. It functions in regulating normal growth and metabolism. Disease involving the thyroid is common but often, particularly in the elderly, the usual signs and symptoms are masked. Diagnosis depends on thyroid function tests of the blood.

Hyperthyroidism occurs when the body is exposed to excessive thyroid hormone. Several forms occur. They all share certain manifestations, such as heat intolerance, increased sweating, and weight loss with increased appetite and food intake. Nervousness, tremors, fatigue, and weakness are common. Muscle weakness with thyroid disease usually is painless and involves primarily the shoulder and pelvic girdle muscles. The shoulders are also involved in a periarthritis similar to that seen in diabetes mellitus. *Chronic Regional Pain Syndrome* also known as *shoulder-hand syndrome* or *reflex sympathetic dystrophy* can occur secondary to this periarthritis. A more generalized loss of bone mass may also be seen. Decreased menses and loss of sexual desire are also found. Palpitations occur with changes in heart rate and cardiac output. With one form of hyperthyroidism called *Graves' disease,* there is a characteristic protuberance of the eyes. Thickening of the skin on the legs (called myxedema) also occurs. This thickening is darker in color and irregular in texture, similar to an orange peel. This thickening can trap the nerve and cause a foot drop with an abnormal sensation on the outer side of the leg *(peroneal neuropathy).* A bone change, called *thyroid acropachy,* rarely occurs in Grave's disease. The surface layer of bone or periosteum becomes inflamed, and bones in the hands and feet thicken. The affected hand or foot may swell, and knee and hip pain can occur.

Hypothyroidism, or underactivity of the thyroid gland, is relatively common, especially in older people. It may follow treatment with radioactive iodine for an overactive gland. More often, an overactive gland burns out, resulting in thyroid underactivity. An underactive gland can occur spontaneously or with an iodine deficiency. Signs of lack of thyroid hormone are diffuse and affect the entire body. Complaints of profound fatigue are common. The skin is cool, coarse, dry, and puffy, with swelling around the eyes. The voice is hoarse and often slow. Complaints of cold intolerance are common, and weight gain, even with decreased food intake, is noted. Constipation and decreased sweating are common.

The heart beat may be slow, and heart enlargement may be found, due to fluid in the sac around the heart. Menses are irregular. Muscle cramps, stiffness, and aching are common. Direct muscle injury is reflected by elevated muscle enzymes found in the blood. Diffuse joint aches and pains occur. Bone resorption and reformation are slow. An arthritis involving hands and feet may occur, mimicking *rheumatoid arthritis.* Calcium deposits *(chondrocalcinosis)* in the joint space, especially in the knees, may be found. The joints have a greater tendency to become inflamed with the crystal disease, a condition called *pseudogout.* However, probably the most significant involvement is neurologic. During the physical examination, reflex testing shows a very characteristic slowing. For example, the knee jerk occurs and is followed by a very slow return. *Carpal tunnel syndrome* and other nerve entrapment syndromes are common. Headaches, seizures, and abnormalities of higher mental function also are found.

Metabolic and Inherited Diseases

High Cholesterol and Triglycerides

Elevated cholesterol or triglycerides is called *hyperlipidemia.* High levels of these blood fats are risk factors for heart disease and artery disease in general. What many people do not realize is that extreme elevations of cholesterol or triglycerides may cause joint pain and inflammation. The joints involved may be the ankle, knee, or the small joints of the hands.

Involvement may also occur in the shoulders, hips, wrists, ankles, and balls of the feet.

The joints may become severely inflamed and swollen. Sedimentation rate, which is a measure of inflammation in the body, may increase. The first toe may swell up as if it were having a gouty episode. The tendons, particularly the Achilles tendon at the heel, may become inflamed. Hyperlipidemia may imitate *rheumatoid arthritis, rheumatic fever, gout,* or almost any inflammatory joint condition. In addition, nodules consisting of the fatty material may occur along tendons or along bones. These may imitate the nodules of rheumatoid arthritis or the tophi of gout. Patients with inflamed or tender joints should have an evaluation of cholesterol and triglycerides to be certain hyperlipidemia is not the culprit.

Hemochromatosis

This genetic defect causes abnormal accumulation of iron in tissues. The iron may concentrate in various organs, producing diabetes (pancreas), liver cirrhosis, or heart failure and rhythm abnormalities. Iron deposition also is seen in the joints, leading to a form of severe and accelerated osteoarthritis with cartilage calcification. Hand involvement is common and occurs early. The most important diagnostic feature is involvement of the second and third knuckles or metacarpophalangeal joints that does not typically occur in the usual form of osteoarthritis. Most importantly, hemochromatosis may be confused with rheumatoid arthritis. In addition, calcium pyrophosphate deposition disease, which can cause pseudogout, is often associated with hemochromatosis.

The excess iron may accumulate in the skin, causing a bronze appearance. The iron may infiltrate and destroy the pituitary gland in the brain, causing a multitude of endocrine problems, including loss of libido.

When hemochromatosis is of long duration, the incidence of liver cancer appears to be increased.

Interestingly, the medieval technique of blood-letting is just the prescription necessary to effectively treat hemochromatosis. By drawing off blood on a weekly or monthly basis, the excess iron stores are depleted, thereby preventing the destructive processes described above.

Ochronosis or Alkaptonuria

Ochronosis is a rare inherited disease that causes abnormal metabolism of certain protein components. This metabolic defect leads to the accumulation of a compound that becomes dark colored on exposure to oxygen or alkali. This material accumulates in the cartilage as well as in the skin and whites of the eyes, giving a characteristic pattern of abnormal coloration. However, the accumulation in cartilage causes more than simple color change. Combination of the pigment with cartilage fibers causes a change in the cartilage matrix and accelerates a process of rapid destruction. The cartilage may become calcified. A particularly destructive process is seen in the spine in the cartilage discs.

Bone and Connective Tissue Diseases

Osteoporosis

Bone is a living tissue, constantly changing and being remodeled. With osteoporosis, bones are weakened because bone resorption occurs faster than bone replacement. This tends to occur naturally with aging. During childhood, bone is being deposited faster than it is resorbed. If a good diet is maintained, from about age 20 to 50 bone formation and resorption occur at about an equal rate and bone density stays relatively constant. After 50, the bone mass naturally begins to decrease—especially after menopause in women. Osteoporosis is therefore a decrease in bone mass. Bone mass includes calcium and the protein matrix upon which it is embedded.

Certain families and ethnic groups seem to have a higher incidence of osteoporosis, suggesting a genetic component. Other factors predisposing to osteoporosis include small frame, low dietary calcium intake, and low vitamin D levels, often from insufficient exposure to sunlight. Smoking, caffeine, and alcohol are also predisposing factors.

Other diseases may be associated with osteoporosis. Poor diet as well as intestinal malabsorption and malnutrition contribute. Lack of activity against gravity and prolonged immobility cause increased bone resorption. Local osteoporosis or bone changes often occur after a cast or other immobilizer is used. Space flight with its loss of gravity also accelerates osteoporosis. Surgical removal of the ovaries also can speed osteoporosis because of lack of estrogen.

Osteoporosis is seen in various endocrine abnormalities—thyroid disease, diabetes, Cushing's syndrome (excess production of the body's own cortisone). It is seen in many patients with rheumatoid arthritis but especially in those taking chronic corticosteroids.

Loss of bone density in osteoporosis is an important cause of pain and disability in the elderly—and indirectly of death. When bones are less dense, fractures may occur spontaneously—without a fall of other trauma. This can cause pain in the hip and often in the thigh. The back also is commonly involved with compression fractures of the vertebral bodies. Acute fractures can cause intense pain, usually in the low or upper back but often radiating around to the chest. Chest pain also is the result of spontaneous rib fractures that may occur with no more trauma than a cough or deep breath. Treatment of these fractures with immobilization often leads to an increased incidence of pneumonia.

Paget's Disease of Bone

This disorder, also called osteitis deformans, is a relatively common disorder of bone remodeling occurring in adults over age 40. Bone undergoes changes daily to maintain structure and strength. Bone resorption is accomplished by bone-destroying cells called osteoclasts. Bone formation and calcium deposition are accomplished by the bone-making cells or osteoblasts. In Paget's disease, there is both an acceleration of the destructive and the reconstructive processes, causing a patchy change in the bones, which may lead to severe deformity and marked local pain.

Structural changes in the skull may occur, causing problems with jaw and dental function. Headaches can then occur. Whooshing sounds occur from increased blood flow to the skull, and hearing loss may result because of involvement of the "hearing bones" or ossicles. Dramatic changes in the long bones may also occur, causing bowing of the legs with marked pain and difficulty walking. Severe pain in the hips, thighs, and lower legs may ensue. The clavicles or the bones across the upper chest may be involved, causing chest pain. Characteristic involvement of the spine and pelvis cause alterations in posture with severe back pain. Spine involvement can cause vertebral breaks called compression fractures, which may squeeze the spinal cord or associated nerves.

The bone produced in Paget's disease is not structurally normal. It appears more fragile; pathologic fractures (breaks) often occur. Because it appears abnormal on X-rays, it is sometimes mistaken for cancer. However, on the other hand, tumor may actually develop in abnormal Pagetic bone late in the disease, although this is rare.

Paget's disease may be accompanied by severe pain at the site of active bony turnover. The pain usually is deep and poorly localized. It will often waken the person at night and responds poorly to pain medications, even narcotics. However, in other patients pain may be minimal or not present at all, even in the presence of severe bone involvement.

Hypertrophic Osteoarthropathy

"Clubbing" of the fingers is the hallmark of this condition. It is manifest by a so-called drumstick deformity, where the nailbed is rounded and boggy and the end of the finger appears enlarged—like a drumstick. This deformity appears to start with swelling and inflammation near the ends of the long bones. As this progresses, the periosteum or surface covering of the bone lifts and new bone forms under it. Bone does not typically grow in this way. Normally it grows at specific sites, in a predetermined pattern, and then generally stops enlarging when maturity is reached. This is not to say that bone is not a living tissue, for bone repair and remodeling go on for life. However, growth patterns are well defined and rarely deviated from unless some disease process is present.

Hypertrophic osteoarthropathy may occur in isolation, usually as an inherited defect, but more commonly seems to be associated with other diseases. It is most often seen with lung cancer, either primary carcinoma or metastatic tumor to the lungs, but may also occur with other problems. Chronic lung infections, cystic fibrosis, congenital heart disease, liver disease, and inflammatory conditions involving the bowel are among some of the more common associations.

The bone deformity in this entity may be entirely asymptomatic but is sometimes very painful, especially when associated with underlying cancer. Pain may occur in the long bones of the arms and fingers, but there is a greater tendency for discomfort in the lower legs.

Marfan's Syndrome

This inherited connective tissue abnormality is associated with skeletal abnormalities and eye, heart, and blood vessel problems.

Patients with Marfan's are very tall with long, spider-like fingers (arachnodactyly). Because of this and increased flexibility, the thumb can actually be laid across the palm inside a closed fist, with the tip of the thumb significantly protruding. The arms are also long, and measurement of fingertip-to-fingertip arm span is actually greater than height. Chest deformity and significant curvature of the spine are also present. Because of increased joint mobility, the incidence of early degenerative joint changes is increased, perhaps from joint injury due to instability. Knee problems also are common.

Cardiovascular manifestations also appear to be the result of connective tissue abnormalities. Aortic aneurysm development and rupture may occur. Heart valve disease involving the aortic and mitral valves also is common.

Eye abnormalities classically include slippage or dislocation of the lens. Nearsightedness may also occur.

Ehlers-Danlos Syndrome

This is an inherited defect in the body's connective tissue. The skin is thin and fragile and may tear easily. Joints are extra flexible, what is sometimes called "double-jointed." These patients may develop joint dislocation, joint deformity, accelerated osteoarthritis and may have a proclivity toward tearing of muscles, tendons and ligaments. Spine deformities, joint and muscle aches are common.

Benign Joint Hypermobility Syndrome

This condition is due to a defect in connective tissue but differs from Marfans and Ehlers-Danlos Syndrome in that it primarily affects the joints. The patient's joints are extremely flexible and many are told that they are "double-jointed." There is no systemic disease. The hypermobile joints are prone to dislocation and early osteoarthritis. The most common complaint is that of joint pain. Any joint may be involved. There is a tendency toward ligament and tendon rupture. Such patients may also suffer from pes planus (flat feet), spine scoliosis (curvature), patella (kneecap) subluxation, and knock knees.

Cardiovascular Diseases

Inflammation of the Blood Vessels (Vasculitis)

Vasculitis is basically an inflammation of the blood vessels. There are many forms of this condition involving various-sized blood vessels and various organs. Vasculitis may occur as part of a connective tissue disease (lupus, rheumatoid arthritis, Sjögren's syndrome, for example), in Giant Cell Arteritis, and a variety of other conditions.

Temporal or Giant Cell Arteritis

Painful inflammation of the medium and large-sized arteries branching from the upper aorta, and particularly those in the temples, may occur in people over age 50. Under the microscope, "giant cells" are found in the inflamed blood vessels. The involved vessels can become blocked, causing damage to the organs to which they supply blood flow. Involvement of the blood vessels feeding the back of the eye can lead to visual loss. Since this visual loss can be permanent, accurate and rapid diagnosis and treatment of this condition is mandatory to avoid potential blindness. Other complications may include stroke and heart attack.

Onset of symptoms may be sudden, but usually the problem develops slowly and is not immediately recognized. Fevers, weight loss, fatigue, and simply "feeling poorly" are often the first signs. Headaches will commonly develop and often there is tenderness over the temporal arteries in the forehead. Pain may also involve the back of the head or upper neck with involvement of the occipital arteries. Generalized scalp tenderness may also be a complaint. Pain in the jaw that worsens with chewing also is common. Permanent visual loss occurs in many patients but is believed preventable with early recognition and treatment. The disease is often associated with another entity called *polymyalgia rheumatica* (PMR). Diagnosis usually is made by biopsy of the involved blood vessel, usually the temporal artery in the temple. Associated laboratory findings usually include anemia or low blood count, mild liver test abnormalities and a high sedimentation rate.

A late complication of giant cell arteritis is the development of aneurysms of arteries. These aneurysms may rupture at a later date, even after the condition is brought under control with medications. Careful follow up after the disease is quiescent is therefore imperative.

Pericarditis

Pericarditis is the usually painful inflammation of the sac surrounding the heart. Chest pain varies with position and often with breathing, swallowing, or yawning. The pain tends to be very sharp and knife-like in character, often worse when lying down. It is usually in the chest but often radiates to the neck or left shoulder or arm. The pericardial inflammation often is accompanied by an effusion, or accumulation of fluid, in the pericardial sac. Under some circumstances, the fluid accumulation is sufficient to interfere with the normal beating of the heart. The extreme of this problem is called cardiac tamponade, which can stop heart function.

Systemic lupus erythematosus often is associated with serositis or inflammation of the sacs surrounding the heart, the lungs, and the intestines. *Drug induced lupus* (caused by medication) seems to frequently be accompanied by a serositis, often with pericarditis. Pericarditis in lupus rarely progresses to severe cardiac compromise and tamponade.
Tuberculosis is another chronic condition associated with pericardial inflammation and effusion.

Pericardial involvement is common in *rheumatoid arthritis* but usually does not cause any problem.

Sometimes pericarditis is not associated with a distinct cause and is termed *idiopathic pericarditis.*

Angina

This is discomfort experienced when heart muscle does not have adequate blood flow. The classic history for angina is pressure beneath the breastbone that may move or radiate to the left shoulder and down the inside of the left arm, even to the fingers. The pain may move to the back, the throat, the jaw and teeth, and sometimes even down the right arm. Angina may even be felt in the upper or lower abdominal area. Interestingly, it seldom occurs on the left side of the chest in front of the heart. Most patients with pain in front of the heart on the left side of the chest do not have angina. Angina sometimes causes unusual symptoms. Hoarseness, jaw pain, and pain in the left arm without any chest pain can signal atypical angina. It is important to consider activities that precipitate or aggravate the pain. Physical activities may increase the heart rate and cause pain which may actually be due to atypical angina. The heart may have very significant narrowing in its blood vessels, and angina may be a warning of impending heart attack.

Peripheral Arterial Disease

"Poor circulation" can occur in either the veins (blood vessels bring blood back to the heart) or arteries (vessels carrying blood away from the heart). Peripheral arterial disease often results from arteriosclerosis, or cholesterol plaque formation, which narrows blood vessels. Discomfort in the legs is most common. The actual problem is a lack of blood supply to exercising muscles, particularly the calf muscles. Patients describe the discomfort as a pain, ache, cramp, or sensation of the legs feeling tired, particularly with walking. Resting often helps by decreasing the oxygen demands and therefore the blood flow needed by the calf muscle. As artery disease advances, patients are less capable of walking. Eventually leg and foot pain may occur even during rest.

Sometimes the blood vessel involvement is higher up where the blood vessels branch off from the main blood vessels to bring blood flow down the legs. When the flow decreases higher up, pain can occur in the buttocks and hips as well as the calves. Sometimes the decreased blood flow is more distant, nearer the foot. The pulses in the involved foot may be diminished. Eventually, if the lack of blood is severe enough, the tissue can die and gangrene can set in.

It is important to consider artery disease in patients with pain in one or both legs while walking. It is important to note that lumbar spinal stenosis symptoms may imitate the symptoms of lower extremity arterial disease. This is called pseudoclaudcation.

Abdominal Aortic Aneurysm

An aneurysm is an enlargement of a blood vessel. When the vessel's diameter increases, the elastic wall becomes thinner, just as happens when a balloon is blown up. Eventually aneurysms cause pain by pressing on other structures, by rupturing (breaking), or by a process called dissection.

273

Dissection occurs when blood flows within the wall of the blood vessel itself, separating the layers of the large artery wall.

An aneurysm in the lower abdomen is called an abdominal aortic aneurysm. When it reaches a critical size, it may cause pressure on the spine, which in turn causes a boring pain into the abdomen or back. This type of pain should be considered a clue to possible aneurysm. The aneurysm may rupture or leak, causing shock and death.

Gastrointestinal Disorders

Reactive Arthritis or *Reiter's Syndrome*

Classic Reiter's syndrome of inflammation of the joints, eyes, and genitals causes typical skin rashes and is generally thought to be a sexually transmitted disease. (It is discussed more extensively elsewhere in this book). However, reactive arthritis also has been documented after bacterially induced gastroenteritis, particularly with Shigella and Salmonella. It appears to be a reactive process triggered by infection in genetically susceptible individuals. This form of post infectious arthritis usually does not respond to treatment with antibiotics.

Post-Intestinal Bypass Syndrome

Intestinal bypass is used as a treatment for severe obesity. Accumulation of bacteria and proteins in the blind, bypassed loop of bowel is believed to trigger an immune reaction. Usually a high circulating level of IgA, an immune protein, is secreted in the gut. As bacterial proteins enter the circulation, the body's proteins combine with them to form immune complexes that can trigger certain reactions. These include a skin rash as well as an arthritis that seems to skip from joint to joint but does not cause deformity. Other organ damage may also occur.

Microbiome

A series of studies from the Mayo Clinic as well as from other institutions has demonstrated that the microbiome or gut bacteria may play a significant role in the development of rheumatoid arthritis and possibly other forms of arthritis as well.

According to a press release from the Mayo Clinic and reported in Eureka, in 2016, "the bacteria in your gut do more than break down your food. They also can predict susceptibility to rheumatoid arthritis, suggests Veena Taneja, Ph.D., an immunologist at Mayo Clinic's Center for Individualized Medicine. Dr. Taneja recently published two studies -- one in *Genome Medicine* and one in *Arthritis and Rheumatology* -- connecting the dots between gut microbiota and rheumatoid arthritis."

Dr. Taneja and her team identified intestinal bacteria as a possible cause; their studies indicate that testing for specific microbiota in the gut can help physicians predict and prevent the onset of rheumatoid arthritis.

"These are exciting discoveries that we may be able to use to personalize treatment for patients," Dr. Taneja says.

Eureka goes on to comment, "the paper published in *Genome Medicine* summarizes a study of rheumatoid arthritis patients, their relatives and a healthy control group. The study aimed to find a biomarker -- or a substance that indicates a disease, condition or phenomena -- that predicts susceptibility to rheumatoid arthritis. They noted that an abundance of certain rare bacterial lineages causes a microbial imbalance that is found in rheumatoid arthritis patients.

"Using genomic sequencing technology, we were able to pin down some gut microbes that were normally rare and of low abundance in healthy individuals, but expanded in patients with rheumatoid arthritis," Dr. Taneja says."

After further research in mice and, eventually, humans, intestinal microbiota and metabolic signatures could help scientists build a predictive profile for who is likely to develop rheumatoid arthritis and the course the disease will take, Dr. Taneja says.

Based on mouse studies, researchers found an association between the gut microbe Collinsella and the arthritis phenotype. The presence of these bacteria may lead to new ways to diagnose patients and to reduce the imbalance that causes rheumatoid arthritis before or in its early stages, according to John Davis III, M.D., and Eric Matteson, M.D., Mayo Clinic rheumatologists and study co-authors. Continued research could lead to preventive treatments.

The second paper, published in *Arthritis and Rheumatology*, explored another facet of gut bacteria. Dr. Taneja treated one group of arthritis-susceptible mice with a bacterium, Prevotella histicola, and compared that to a group that had no treatment. The study found that mice treated with the bacterium had decreased symptom frequency and severity, and fewer inflammatory conditions associated with rheumatoid arthritis. The treatment produced fewer side effects, such as weight gain and villous atrophy -- a condition that prevents the gut from absorbing nutrients -- that may be linked with other, more traditional treatments.

While human trials have not yet taken place, the mice's immune systems and arthritis mimic humans, and shows promise for similar, positive effects. Since this bacterium is a part of healthy human gut, treatment is less likely to have side effects, says study co-author Joseph Murray, M.D., a Mayo Clinic gastroenterologist.

Tumors Involving Bones and Joints

Cancerous tumors may cause bone and joint aches and pain three ways. The malignant (cancerous) tumor can originate in the bones or joints. Secondly, a metastatic tumor might be found in the bones and joints, having spread from another distant primary tumor. Finally, bone and joint aches and pains may arise from so-called *paraneoplastic syndrome,* where various symptoms are caused by a distant primary tumor.

Primary malignancies of the bones and joints account for only a small proportion of all cancerous tumors. Usually the symptoms include severe local pain and an unusual lump or swelling. These occur primarily in the younger person and are diagnosed with X-rays and special studies, including bone scans. When malignancy is suspected, based on noninvasive studies, a biopsy must be done to specifically define the kind of tissue involved. Any site can be affected but legs are most often involved. Other areas include hips, knees, shoulders, chest, and lower and upper back.

Secondary or metastatic tumors are especially common in the older person. Sometimes bone or joint pain is the first sign of a distant primary tumor. When bone metastases are found in a person with a strong family history of breast cancer, this primary tumor should be searched for aggressively. In an older man with a change in urinary habits, a primary prostate cancer should be sought. Lung, kidney, and thyroid cancers and a blood malignancy called myeloma also commonly involve bone.

Although metastatic cancer can affect almost any bone, prostate cancer and myeloma tend to involve the low back and breast cancer the upper back and chest. Back involvement may mimic the compression fractures seen in osteoporosis. Lung cancer sometimes involves the small bones of the hand.

Paraneoplastic Syndromes

Paraneoplastic syndromes are symptoms caused by effects of remote tumors. The symptoms are not due to the direct spread of the tumor but may be mediated by chemicals produced by the tumor or in response to the tumor. These syndromes can affect all body systems and may be the first clue to cancer.

The most common symptoms of cancer may be well known—fever, weight loss, and abnormalities of metabolism, such as high blood calcium levels. Other paraneoplastic manifestations might include aches and pains in locations far off from the tumor itself. For example, the rapid onset of arthritis in an elderly person may be associated with an underlying hidden cancer. The arthritis may seem to be rheumatoid arthritis and yet *rheumatoid nodules* in the skin and *rheumatoid factor* in the blood are not present. Hopefully, the underlying tumor is detected. Treatment of the primary cancer relieves the arthritis symptoms, and conversely the arthritis returns if the tumor regrows after therapy.

Muscle abnormalities also may occur in association with cancer. *Dermatomyositis* and less frequently *polymyositis*, which cause inflammatory destruction of muscle, are associated with malignancy in as many as 20 percent of cases. *Carcinomatous myopathy* is the name given to other muscle abnormalities that differ from dermatomyositis or polymyositis. Muscle wasting and weakness are prominent features. All of these muscle abnormalities appear to regress when the tumor is treated and frequently return if the tumor regrows.

What are the clues to malignancy in association with aches and pains? Usually the involved person is older. Pain, distribution of involved areas, and other signs are not typical of connective tissue disease. The pain often is severe, frequently occurring at night and waking the person. The onset of symptoms is usually explosive and often involves unexpected locations. Finally, and most important, there are clues to underlying disease. Sometimes a mass is felt, or maybe there is blood in a bowel movement or when coughing. Perhaps a new hoarseness or a change in bowel habits has occurred. These minor symptoms are often a call for you to pay extra attention to your body. If cancer is discovered, early detection will greatly increase the chance of cure.

Multiple Myeloma

Uncontrolled cell growth of a plasma cell that produces a specific protein secreted into the blood is the main characteristic of myeloma. These plasma cells are located in the bone marrow and can cause painful bone marrow tumors. These usually occur in the spine, chest, and pelvis and can be single or multiple. This form of cancer may be associated with joint pain, weakness, fatigue, anemia, infection (especially pneumonia), kidney failure, and spontaneous breaks in bones.

Miscellaneous Conditions

Kidney Stones

Formation of stones in the urinary system occurs in various ways. Once formed, a stone may block the ureter or tubing between the kidney and bladder. This causes renal colic, a severe pain that usually occurs in waves. The pain is located in the low back, usually just below the ribs. Pain may be referred around the flank and into the groin down to the genitals. It is often mistakenly attributed to a "bad hip."

Calcium stones occur when calcium concentrations in urine are high. This commonly occurs in *sarcoidosis,* as well as with overproduction of parathyroid hormone *(hyperparathyroidism).* Calcium stones are also sometimes found with excessive calcium intake from milk or certain antacids. Excess vitamin D also may contribute to stone formation. Intestinal bypass surgery is a cause of kidney stone formation in some patients; this is due to relative dehydration and elevated oxalate levels.

Eosinophilia Myalgia Syndrome (EMS)

In the late 1980s, the drug L-tryptophan, a nonprescription sleep promoter, was found to cause a number of strange symptoms. The syndrome included muscle and joint pain, elevated allergic eosinophils in the blood, and tightening and thickening of the skin. The skin thickening resembled progressive systemic sclerosis *(scleroderma)* but lacked the typical finger changes and Raynaud's phenomena (extreme discomfort when fingers or toes are exposed to cold).

Fever, pneumonia, nerve and heart problems, abnormal liver tests, and a variety of rashes also have been associated with use of L-tryptophan. A number of patients were quite ill and required high-dose cortisone. Not all improved.

The disorder was found to be caused by L-tryptophan made by a single

279

Japanese company. However, since then, L-tryptophan has been taken off the market. Despite the passage of time, a number of patients did not improve. Different treatments had been tried in an attempt to suppress the immune system and alleviate symptoms.

The situation with EMS suggests exposure to a chemical may alter the body's immune system. Also, the effects can be permanent or long lasting, well beyond the time the chemical would be expected to remain in the body. A number of other medications and chemicals have caused thickening of the skin resembling *scleroderma*. Among them are adulterated rape seed oil, silica and silicone, vinyl chloride, bleomycin (a chemotherapy drug), organic solvents, epoxy resins, bromocriptine, phytonadione, pentazocine, certain appetite suppressants, and cocaine.

Baker's Cyst

A Baker's cyst (popliteal cyst) occurs when fluid from the knee moves into a bursa behind the knee, causing swelling. These cysts occur in almost any condition that damages a knee. *Rheumatoid arthritis, internal derangement of the knees,* and *osteoarthritis* can lead to cyst formation. Any chronic knee arthritis may result in a Baker's cyst.

The cyst can dissect (spread down the leg into the calf). This can resemble thrombophlebitis or an inflamed and clotted vein. The cyst may rupture into the calf and cause very significant pain.

Baker's cysts cause discomfort primarily in the back of the knee. Treatment consists of injection of steroids into the knee and correction of the underlying knee disorder when necessary. Ultrasound needle guidance can be used to safely evacuate the fluid and inject glucocorticoid. Also, the presence of a Baker's cyst should not dissuade the clinician from looking for the presence of a concomitant blood clot.

Kyphosis

Kyphosis is the medical name for a humped or hunched back. It is different from scoliosis, which is more of an "S" curvature of the spine. Kyphosis may occur with scoliosis.

The most common cause is *osteoporosis* or thinning of the bone, particularly in elderly women. This is sometimes called *dowager's hump.* The usually square-shaped bones of the spine (vertebrae) thin and wedge in front, causing the chest to cave in. This wedging may be sudden (osteoporotic compression fracture) or it may be gradual. Fractures often result in muscle spasm and pain that radiates or moves around the chest wall toward the front. Height is decreased and the ability to take a deep breath is compromised. The lower front ribs often are brought down toward the pelvic bones. Because it is difficult for these people to take a deep breath, the incidence of pneumonia is increased. Chronic back pain may occur, but some patients have no significant discomfort.

One form of kyphosis occurs in teenagers or young adults and is called juvenile kyphosis of Scheuermann's disease. The cause is probably an abnormality of the bony vertebrae in the spine. Many of these young patients describe mid-back pain and have a history of having "slouched" for many years. The cause of Scheuermann's disease is unknown. The condition is treated by exercise and sometimes by bracing. If the deformity is severe, surgery may be needed.

Chronic Fatigue Syndrome (CFS)

The concept of chronic fatigue syndrome or even the existence of a specific syndrome causing fatigue has evolved over the past 50 years. Epidemics of severe fatigue and weakness have been described as *"neuromyasthenia."* These epidemics seem to be isolated to certain localities and were basically unexplained or sometimes attributed to "mass hysteria." In the 1980s, there has been a growing awareness of many patients, especially young women, who have severe debilitating fatigue. This fatigue initially was attributed to a persistent *Epstein-Barr virus infection* because many of these patients had high antibody levels against this virus. However, studies showed that the high antibody titers were not exclusive to these patients. The name chronic *Epstein-Barr viral syndrome* was then changed to chronic fatigue syndrome.

An important attribute of many CFS patients is immune system dysfunction. The immune system may be "up-regulated," producing excessive antibodies and being "turned on" even without infection. In other patients, the immune system is faulty; these patients have an increased number of infections, especially respiratory infections.

It is the sentiment of some physicians that many of these patients are simply depressed. It is difficult to make that assumption when a person who has been quite active suddenly finds himself or herself with severe fatigue. That alone could lead to depression. Likewise, it was believed by some that many of these patients suffered from an underlying infection that was poorly delineated, such as chronic *brucellosis,* systemic *candidiasis, postpolio syndrome,* and *Lyme disease.* Most, however, have been shown to not have any of these specific conditions.

The symptoms of chronic fatigue syndrome, aside from the debilitating fatigue, are many. Among them are fever, sore throat, painful nodes, muscle weakness, muscle pain, headaches, joint pain, difficulty looking at light, decreased ability to concentrate, confusion, and sleep disturbances. Many other symptoms have been described by these patients.

Diagnosis of chronic fatigue syndrome requires elimination of many conditions that can cause fatigue. These include tumors, connective tissue diseases, certain other infections (including Lyme disease, tuberculosis, parasite infections, and AIDS, to name a few). Other conditions that must be ruled out are chronic hepatitis, sarcoidosis, major depression, sleep disorders, nerve or muscle diseases, endocrine diseases, medication side effects, and other chronic diseases of the heart, lung, gastrointestinal tract, kidney, and bone marrow. No specific tests are available for chronic fatigue syndrome. Therefore, diagnosis involves exclusion of other conditions that could be responsible.

Some researchers believe chronic fatigue syndrome is caused by a poorly identified retrovirus. Much research is in progress to help identify this agent.

Many people with chronic fatigue syndrome have fibromyalgia. (Please see the separate section of this book for more detail on this condition.) With fibromyalgia, sleep is not refreshing, leading to chronic fatigue, muscle and joint aches, depression, chronic pain, and development of painful areas called trigger points. These points are often in the back and neck. Fibromyalgia is treatable to a certain degree. Medications can be used to improve sleep, alleviate depression, and reduce inflammation. Physical therapy also is sometimes helpful.

Treatment of chronic fatigue syndrome is, at best, frustrating. As a general rule of thumb, one-third of the patients defined as having this condition improve fairly rapidly over several months. Another third improve to some degree over a period of years. The final third will not improve at all and may even become worse.

The most effective treatment involves alleviating the fibromyalgia present in most CFS patients. Other treatment plans include a trial of acyclovir (an antiviral medication), gamma-globulin injections, vitamin B12 injections, calcium channel blockers, opiate receptor blockers, and other medications, depending on the symptoms. To date, no specific treatment has met with resounding success. Treatment is usually supportive and aimed at the underlying symptoms.

Chronic fatigue syndrome remains controversial. Not all physicians are convinced that it exists as a distinct entity. A great deal of knowledge needs to be acquired regarding its cause and treatment.

Enlarged Neck Nodes

These nodes, also called lymph nodes, are aggregates of white blood cells that help produce an immune response to infection and tumor. Lymph nodes may enlarge because of an increase in the number of white cells responding to a foreign protein, inflammatory conditions, by the transformation of white blood cells into tumor cells as in lymphoma, the movement of cancer cells from another organ into the lymph nodes, and with the occurrence of certain metabolic conditions.

Connective tissue diseases such as *rheumatoid arthritis* and *lupus,* certain drugs, AIDS, various infections, and certain inflammatory disease may cause lymph node enlargement. Nodes may be painless or painful. Painless enlargement may be associated with inflammatory conditions as well as with tumors. Painful enlargement often is associated with infection. However, this rule is not clear-cut.

The back of the neck may develop lymph node enlargement because of a variety of virus infections, *toxoplasmosis* (a protozoan parasite), and *syphilis.* In addition, a number of tumors may be associated with enlarged lymph nodes in the back of the neck.

Lymph node enlargement in the front of the neck often is due to infection. Such infection may be in the sinuses or in the teeth.

Certainly any neck lymph node may enlarge due to infection, including AIDS, drug reactions, inflammatory and connective tissue diseases, and tumors. The enlarged nodes may be a cause of discomfort and need to be thoroughly investigated, particularly if the node has been enlarged for an extended period of time.

Fixed Sacroiliac Joint Syndrome

The sacroiliac joints are paired joints located at the bottom of the low back, near the inner and upper areas of the buttocks. These joints normally have some movement. Sometimes the sacroiliac joint on one side becomes locked after a fall onto the buttocks or a twisting motion. The patient may feel a dull pain on one side of the low back in the buttocks area. This may move into the groin or to the front of the thigh or even down the leg, imitating *sciatica.* The low back is tender on the side of the fixed or locked sacroiliac joint. The leg on the involved side may feel tired or heavy.

For years the fixed sacroiliac joint had been evaluated and treated only by chiropractors. With time, other health care professionals have come to appreciate the value of mobilization or "manipulation" of the joint to reestablish movement. Treatment is usually effective once the condition is properly diagnosed. A fixed sacroiliac joint can imitate sciatica, many low back conditions, and hip and pelvic pain.

Enlarged Parotid Glands

The parotid glands are in front of the ears, near the jaw. They produce saliva. The parotid glands may enlarge painlessly, such as in mumps, *sarcoidosis,* or tumor. Occasionally these glands become swollen and painful with infection, salivary duct stones, or *Sjögren's syndrome.* Sjögren's syndrome is called dry eye and dry mouth syndrome and occurs when the tear glands and salivary glands become inflamed and function poorly. The parotid gland may be enlarged with or without pain in Sjögren's syndrome. Eventually much of the parotid gland is destroyed, and the mouth becomes dry because very little saliva is produced.

INDEX

A

B

C

Printed in Great Britain
by Amazon